Smile!

Creating Healthy and Beautiful Smiles with Cosmetic Dentistry

Smile!

Creating Healthy and Beautiful Smiles with Cosmetic Dentistry

Blue Ocean Publishing Group

Dunedin, FL

Smile!
Creating Healthy and Beautiful Smiles with Cosmetic Dentistry

Published by Blue Ocean Publishing Group
1497 Main St., Ste 236
Dunedin, FL 34698

ISBN: 978-1-947436-03-9

Library of Congress Control Number: 2020913650

Dedication

This book is dedicated to you, the reader,
because by picking up this book,
you show you care about your oral health.

Table of Contents

INTRODUCTION

This book discusses the benefits of cosmetic dentistry and so much more. It is a resource for you, the patient and the consumer, so that you can learn more about various cosmetic procedures and what they will do for your overall health and well-being. *Smile! Creating Healthy and Beautiful Smiles with Cosmetic Dentistry* will help you understand the complex world of cosmetic dentistry so that you can make informed decisions about your oral treatments.

As a dental patient, you have the right to know what procedures are best for you; the risks and benefits of any dental procedure; the cost of all procedures and if insurance will cover part or all of the expense; and what type of outcome you can reasonably expect from the procedure. Unfortunately, many patients are hesitant to ask questions and even worse, are subjected to high-pressure sales pitches designed only to sell expensive dental work by the doctors they should be able to trust.

This book was created to help you understand all the options you have when faced with choices about your oral care. The experts that have contributed to this book have done so because they want patients to understand these procedures. They also want to allow them to make the right decisions about their own healthcare.

Cosmetic dentistry is not a new practice. Archaeological evidence shows that as early as 700 B.C., dentures were made from ivory and bone. Since then, technological advances through the centuries have increased the popularity of cosmetic dental procedures. Certainly, people throughout the ages have recognized the importance of strong teeth; many cultures have also placed a premium on a beautiful smile. The significance of a healthy, attractive smile has never been more important than it is in today's culture. Because of new technology, particularly made possible by the use of computers, you can have the smile of your dreams, provided that you know which procedures will give you the best outcome.

Today, patients are faced with a vast array of cosmetic dental procedures. In fact, there are so many dental procedures available now that it may be overwhelming to consider all the options. Dentists offer services such as:

- Smile Makeovers
- Crowns
- Teeth Whitening
- Periodontal Treatment
- Veneers
- Dentures
- Bridges
- Implants
- Orthodontics
- Treating incorrect bite

Patients of any age, from the very old to the very young, can safely receive most dental treatments. There is even sedation dentistry for those who suffer from extreme anxiety about dental procedures or for those who simply want a more comfortable experience.

In *Smile! Creating Healthy and Beautiful Smiles with Cosmetic Dentistry*, ten leading dentists from around the country educate you, the reader, about subjects related to cosmetic dentistry. Each of these experts is recognized as a successful leader in their various fields. In this book you will have access to their knowledge and insight on the following topics:

The Importance of a Healthy Attractive Smile – Mary Azadeh Afzali, DDS, offers insight into how important it really is to have a beautiful smile (hint: it may be more important than you think!)

Crowns... They're Not Just for Royalty – Ricardo Zambito, DDS, discusses the importance of crowns and fillings in today's cosmetic dentistry landscape

Brighten Your Smile with Teeth Whitening – Nekia Staley-Neither, DDS, discusses the problem of dull, yellow teeth and how to correct it

The Foundation of a Great Smile – Bryan Kalish, DDS, MS, explains why gum health is the key to overall oral health

Dental Veneers: The Power of Transformation – Steven Davidowitch, DDS, talks about dental veneers and how they can give instant results in brightening and straightening a smile

Biting Right is Biting Tight– Mariana Conant, DDS, helps you understand why your bite is so critical to your overall health and how to make it perfect so you can enjoy years of healthy teeth and gums

Let's Get Something Straight: Orthdontics – Randy Feldman, DDS, MS, explains the facts regarding braces, including both traditional and Invisalign methods

The Consequences of Missing Teeth – Alexander Rockwell, DMD, discusses the health concerns regarding missing teeth and how this problem can be solved

Filling the Gaps with Dental Implants – James R. Green, DMD, helps you understand how dental implants work and whether they are a good choice for you

Leading the Way with Digital Dentistry – Curtis Hayes, DDS, goes over the new technology advances in dentistry that help achieve better and safer results.

Finally, feel free to jump from one section to another in the book; you do not have to read the chapters in order. Pick your favorite topic and start learning immediately about the things you need to know to make great decisions about your dental care!

Smile! Creating Healthy and Beautiful Smiles with Cosmetic Dentistry is your guide to making the right choices for your own oral health. Let our experts help you make the right decisions about your dental care!

The Advantages of a Beautiful Smile

Having a beautiful smile is important. It affects everything in our life—from our personal confidence to our success at work. Our smile says a lot about us. It's one of the first indicators of our health and fitness, our socio-economic status, our habits, and our personality.

Our physical appearance affects our interactions with others from the time we're born (prettier babies get more attention from caregivers, according to research) to our adult years, influencing our dating behaviors, careers, financial success, marriage, and even how supposedly "impartial" judges and juries rule for or against us in the courtroom. One of the primary factors in determining the perception of human beauty is our smile.

From ancient Greece throughout the modern tradition of Western society, beauty hasn't only been the center of philosophical preoccupation but has been associated with harmony and virtue. There are two striking quotes from Plato about beauty. The first is from one of his dialogues, in which Socrates states, "For measure and symmetry are beauty and virtue all the world over." The other is from *The Republic*: "Ugliness and discord and inharmonious motion are nearly allied to ill worth and ill nature, as grace and harmony are the twin sisters of goodness and virtue and bear their likeness."

When we smile, we're viewed as more attractive and sociable. As a result, an individual who has an engaging smile creates a better energy wherever they go. People feel at ease and happier around them, and people who smile more are more likely to get promoted.

A beautiful smile is a source of personal confidence, and it also projects that confidence to others. It creates a ripple effect that manifests as being liked by others, creating a positive environment, and increasing the chances of achieving personal success. A smile is an amazing source of good energy that continuously generates more and more positive energy around us.

Not only is a beautiful smile aesthetically pleasing, it actually affects our mental and physical health. Smiling affects chemicals released in the body that influence our overall health, from our psychological wellbeing to our immune system.

I'd like to share a story to demonstrate what a profound affect a healthy and beautiful smile can have on someone's life. It was a Wednesday afternoon in September 2019. A lovely lady came into my office. She had given up on the idea of having a beautiful smile, because she was told by every dentist she'd consulted that surgery was the only solution to the skeletal disharmony in her upper jaw.

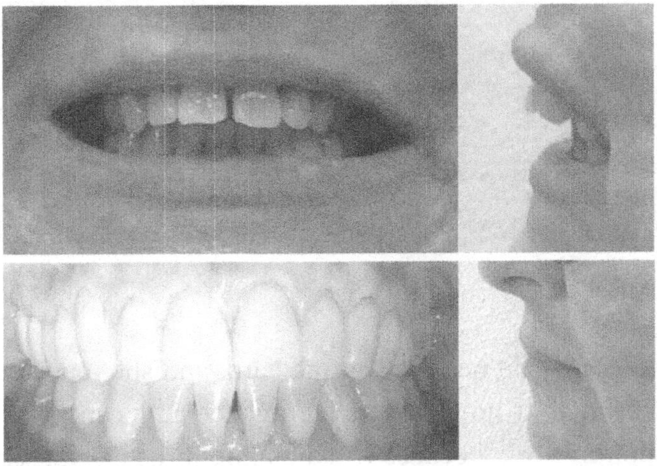

Once I examined her, I identified the issues preventing her from reaching her desired goal of having a beautiful smile. She had a V-shaped palate with both vertical and horizontal bone deficiencies that resulted in the upper jaw protruding significantly and a sixteen-millimeter overjet (a horizontal misalignment between the upper and lower front teeth). This meant her upper teeth were sixteen millimeters in front of her lower teeth, and she had a large, open gap between her upper and lower teeth.

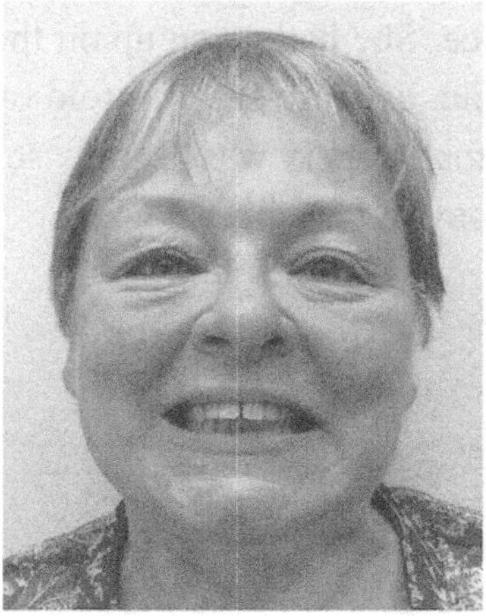

Before

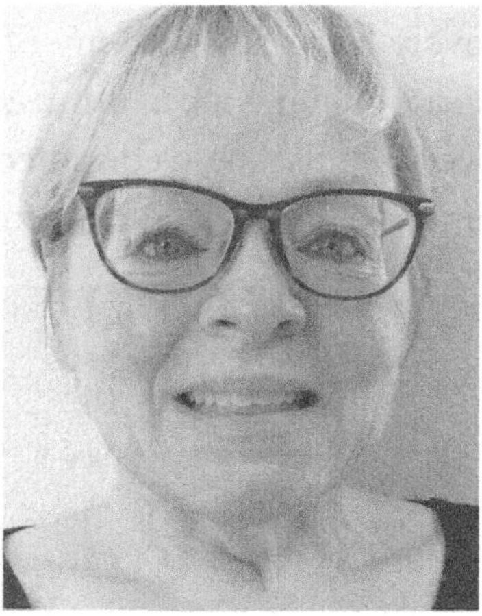

After

The despair in her eyes hit me hard, and she repeated, "I've been told no one can fix my teeth. I can't have orthodontic work, because I'm a tongue-thruster. Surgery is the only solution, and I don't want to have a surgery."

I told her, "I'd love to help you, and I can help you."

I started her orthodontic treatment in September 2019 and completed it in April 2020. After the work was completed, this patient gave a testimonial about her experience with me: "I feel like a new person. I no longer need my CPAP machine to breathe and sleep at night. I lost one hundred pounds, I feel great, and I'm thrilled with my smile."

Why People Don't Smile

One of the main reasons that people don't smile is because they feel their smile actually detracts from their appearance, and this embarrasses them. Maybe they're concerned that their teeth aren't white enough or that they're crooked. Some people are sensitive about the alignment of their teeth, or they have excessive spaces or gaps between their teeth, and this is why they don't smile. Others may have broken teeth or teeth that have been worn down by grinding them. Some may have missing teeth and believe the black holes where the teeth should be are all that people see when they smile. In other cases, restorative efforts—caps, for example—have degraded and are no longer attractive.

Factors such as an overbite or the top teeth not aligning correctly with the bottom teeth can affect the appearance of our smile. This latter condition is called poor occlusion. Occlusion refers to how our upper teeth meet with our lower teeth when we bring them together. The upper teeth need to land correctly on the lower teeth to create an impression of harmony in the smile.

Lastly, the individual may have dentures that don't fit right, and they're worried they may slip or move. As a result, the person is reluctant to smile.

However, all of these detriments to a beautiful smile can be corrected, and that's what I'll be talking about in this chapter.

Two Keys to a Beautiful Smile

What constitutes a beautiful smile is different for each individual, although there are objective factors, as we've mentioned above, that influence whether a smile is perceived as beautiful. However, there are two keys that are essential in determining the beauty of a smile—harmony and functionality.

Aesthetic dentistry is all about creating a harmonious, functional smile. A beautiful smile is not only harmonious with the rest of the facial features but complements the individual's personality.

Such a smile is also functional, which means there's good occlusion—there's a proper relationship of the upper teeth and lower teeth, the incisors to the canines, the canines to the premolars, the premolars to molars, and the upper jaw and lower jaw so the smile and the face are perceived to have harmonious symmetry.

Functionality is essential, because it's possible to invest thousands of dollars in whitening the teeth or some other cosmetic procedure, but, if the basic functionality isn't there, these efforts won't result in the harmony that creates a beautiful smile. This lack of harmony affects the neuromuscular system of the face, which, in turn, influences not only our smile but the appearance of our entire face. In other words, we must begin with the alignment of the upper and lower jaw in creating a beautiful smile.

The Physiological Effects of a Beautiful Smile

Our mouth isn't an isolated entity. It's the gateway to our overall health. It communicates directly with our digestive system and affects the health of our entire body.

The digestive process begins with chewing and with the enzymes in our saliva that initiate the breakdown of food. The mouth is also the breeding ground for bacteria on our teeth, gums, tongue, and other tissues that harbor toxins. Bacteria and toxins from our mouth travel throughout our body and cause problems.

The Immune System

Everything that happens in the body is interconnected. A strong immune system begins with the good oral flora ("good bacteria") in our mouth. If there are too many harmful germs, bacteria, and viruses in our mouth, this compromises our overall immunity. When toxins in the mouth enter our digestive system, they're transferred to the stomach and then the small intestine.

The small intestine plays a large role in our immunity. Our gut is a major part in our immune system, and it's populated with normal flora also known as microbiomes, which are essential for us to maintain our health. One of the most important things to be aware of is that the oral and gut microbiomes are interactively connected. That means, if we're experiencing oral issues (cavities, bleeding gums, periodontal disease, oral thrush, etc.), there's a very good chance that our gut microbiomes are out of balance.

When infectious oral bacteria disturb our healthy gut flora, this creates an imbalance in our immune system that can lead to infections and even serious illness. Research has shown that these inflammatory aspects may contribute to diseases such as cancer, diabetes, Alzheimer's disease, and many other chronic diseases. Chronic inflammation throughout the body, including the brain, can begin in the oral cavity, and poor mouth health directly affects our immune system.

Systemic Inflammation

As many as 80% of Americans have gum disease, which is caused by the accumulation of bacteria in the gums that leads to the formation of plaque and inflammation throughout the body. The bacteria in the mouth produce the same type of plaque that accumulates in the arteries of our heart as well as in arteries throughout our body. This build-up of plaque is called arteriosclerosis, which can cause a heart attack if the plaque is in the arteries of the heart or dementia if the plaque creates blockages in the arteries of the brain.

The presence of bacteria around the gums first results in the deterioration of the gum tissue, causing the gums to recede. Then the toxins from the bacteria erode the bone around the teeth, which leads to the teeth becoming loose and eventually being lost. This, in turn, contributes to loss of function and disharmony in the mouth. Ill-fitting crowns, bridges, and loose filling are all traps that collect bacteria, creating toxins that can affect many places in the body and lead to chronic inflammation.

I tell my patients that the mouth is the center between their brain and their heart. Toxins created by bacteria in the mouth travel up to the brain and down to the heart.

These two vital organs and all the other organs—lungs, liver, pancreas, stomach, everything—are affected.

The Digestive System

Anything that affects our ability to chew—the first, critical step in the digestive process—affects our health. Whether it be ill-fitting dentures or partials, missing teeth, teeth that have been ground down and have lost their sharpness and their efficiency, this all affects the first step of digestion.

Improperly chewed food arrives at the stomach for the second step of the digestive process without being sufficiently prepared, and this can lead to problems such as inflammation. The inability to chew easily often results in people not eating a balanced diet—particularly one that includes fruits and vegetables, which are so vital to our overall health.

In addition to losing the enjoyment we derive from eating the kinds of foods we like and not eating a balanced diet because chewing has become difficult, chewing stimulates the neuromuscular system of the face and keeps the face looking young and animated.

Crooked Teeth

Another contributor to poor mouth health is crooked teeth. Crooked teeth aren't functional, and they also cause gum disease. Plaque is more likely to accumulate between crooked teeth, which are caused by deficiencies in the bone of the jaw. Recent research has shown that there are certain gum bacteria that reside in hollow areas of the jawbone, and these bacteria are resistant to any type of treatment.

A patient may have many deep-cleaning treatments, but the bacteria are never permanently removed because they're harbored in the structural defects in the jawbone. Crooked teeth are a manifestation of those fundamental defects in the jawbone.

Crooked teeth also cause recession of the gums, because the teeth are competing for the same space, and that puts pressure on the gums. There's disharmony in the bite, which puts additional pressure on the gums, leading to recession.

Besides not being attractive or functional, crooked teeth diminish other aesthetics of the smile. Even if a person has very white teeth, if those teeth are crooked, the reflection of light from the enamel is less, and this creates a smile that isn't perceived as bright. The individual believes they need more whitening, but what's actually called for is orthodontic work to straighten the teeth, so they maximally reflect light.

Teeth Grinding

Grinding of the teeth is often associated with crooked teeth because of the disharmony in the bite. Grinding can begin a downward spiral of enamel loss, sensitivity to and inability to tolerate certain foods, lack of interest in eating, and resultant poor nutrition. Ground-down teeth make chewing difficult, which inhibits digestion, affects facial muscle tone, and exacerbates the appearance of aging in the face. Grinding not only causes loss of the surface of the teeth, which results in poor occlusion, but can lead to the loss of the entire tooth. Grinding creates greater disharmony, and this affects the neuromuscular system. As grinding continues, there's loss of tooth structure and, potentially, loss of the teeth themselves.

Enamel is the second strongest material in the body after bones. Mother Nature has fashioned the enamel on our teeth into pointy surfaces on our back teeth and sharp edges on our front teeth so we can tear and chew food. When that protective layer of enamel becomes ground down and thin, this exposes the dentin beneath it, which is softer and deteriorates much faster than enamel. When this happens, the efficiency of our ability to chew decreases drastically, and this initiates another vicious cycle. If it takes a person five years to lose the enamel on their teeth, once the dentin is exposed, they can lose the tooth mass they lost in five or ten years in just a year or two.

As teeth become more and more ground down, they develop sensitivity, and the person begins to avoid certain foods. Usually, people initially become sensitive to cold foods such as ice cream or ice water, because it causes a shooting pain in the tooth that can last for seconds or much longer. Sometimes, just breathing cold air can cause pain in the teeth. The teeth may develop sensitivity to acidic foods such as lemon juice, tomatoes, and coffee, as well.

This sensitivity—and the resulting pain—only increases as more dentin is exposed. Eventually, the pulp, which is in the interior of the tooth, is exposed. The pulp is where the nerves and blood supply are located. If the pulp becomes inflamed and that inflammation continues, it can create an irreversible situation in which the person must undergo a root canal.

Addressing crooked teeth and grinding early can prevent the individual from going through the unnecessarily ordeal of enamel loss, progressive sensitivity, dentin loss, inflammation of the tooth pulp, and the need for a root canal. It all comes back to creating harmony in the bite to keep the neuromuscular system healthy.

Smiling Keeps Us Looking Young and Affects our Mental Health

Believe it or not, smiling affects the physiological aging of our face. Never smiling and making an effort to keep the lips closed affects the facial muscles in the lower face—from just below the nose to the chin. Not using these muscles to smile can cause them to lose tone and droop. The nasolabial folds (the natural indentations that travel from the outside of the nostrils to the corners of the lips) become more pronounced and form deep lines, which makes the person look older.

Smiling gives our facial muscles a workout, and this enhances our ability to chew, speak, laugh, and show expression. When we don't smile, we lose muscle tone and the appearance of our face begins to deteriorate.

In an effort to look younger, people spend a lot of time, energy, and money on a variety of cosmetic procedures, but all they need is to become more comfortable with their smile, so they smile more. Not smiling is the fastest way to promote facial aging. When people look serious, it makes them feel more serious, and the worry they experience because of being self-conscious about their smile creates a vicious cycle of looking older and being worried about looking older, which promotes aging.

Also, when we don't smile, this has an effect on the people in our environment. They may feel we don't like them or we're constantly grumpy, which leads to them not engaging with us. As a result, we become isolated, which can lead to a sense of exclusion and even depression.

Something as basic as feeling our smile isn't attractive can cause clinical depression, which can lead to seeing a psychiatrist or psychologist and taking harmful medications to treat that depression. Unfortunately, these medications not only don't address the real problem but make our oral health much worse due to side effects such as dry mouth, which leads to rampant decay. Caries caused by dry mouth are especially destructive, because the decay attacks the root of the tooth first. These caries are the most difficult to control and often lead to tooth loss.

A beautiful smile isn't all about aesthetics—it's a consideration of all of the above. A bite that's not aligned can cause crooked teeth, crooked teeth can cause gum problems, and gum problems can lead to missing teeth or inflammation and illness throughout the body. The aesthetics of our smile are intimately connected to our physical and mental health.

Two Case Studies

About four years ago, a 40-year-old singer came into my office with an emergency dental situation. He was a tall, handsome man, but he looked exhausted. We talked, and he told me he was very frustrated with the condition of his mouth. He had chronic infections and was often in pain, starting to lose teeth, and having difficulty sleeping as a result. The worst part of it, for him, was that he wanted to record his music and perform, but his oral health was preventing that. My assessment was that he was a grinder.

Dealing with this chronic situation had zapped the energy he needed to devote to his career, plus, the loss of teeth ruined his confidence about his smile and about presenting himself in public. When I saw how the health of his mouth was having such an impact on his life and his career, that was a defining and emotional moment for me in terms of my purpose.

That patient was treated for the infection to restore the health of his gums and teeth. He then received cosmetic dentistry including implants. He's now released an album, and he performed at our most recent Christmas party. This man is now traveling and promoting his music.

Another patient came into my office with excruciating TMJ (temporomandibular joint) pain. She was experiencing a sharp pain in her jaw near her ears. This was a beautiful young lady who worked as a pharmacist, and she was desperate. “This pain is killing me,” she said, “and I've been told I need surgery on my jaw or to have Botox injections in those muscles to relieve the pain.” Also, because her jaw muscles were very tight, her smile was contracted.

My associate examined her and asked my opinion before referring her to an oral surgeon for surgery. We looked at her X-rays, and I said to my associate, “Do you see how her bite isn’t aligned. That’s what is causing her pain.”

The patient said she was skeptical that this was the cause of her problem. She didn't want surgery, but she trusted me, so she let me treat her. Using an advanced orthodontic technique called FASTBRACES®, I was able to correct her bite. She reported to me that, in a matter of three or four days, the pain was gone, and it hasn’t come back. She’s been wearing braces for about four months, and she’ll be out of them soon.

There’s a unity to this process. When you start relaxing the temporomandibular joint by unloading the forces on it, the muscles begin to relax. When they’re not fired up and tense anymore, the face starts looking better and the smile becomes more natural. And, of course, correcting the alignment allows the teeth to show more because the smile is wider.

My patients don't have dark triangles at the corners of their mouth when they smile, which I feel is unaesthetic. Bringing harmony to their upper and lower jaw and restoring function brightens their smile, because a wider smile provides more opportunity for the reflection of light.

The lives of this woman and other professional people are affected adversely by problems like TMJ. The technique that I use is amazing, because the technology is so effective that I've been able get results very, very quickly.

What Makes a Good Cosmetic Dentist?

When choosing a cosmetic dentist, the patient should be educated about dental health, and they need to feel assured that the doctor has an understanding of the neuromuscular system, the bite, and aesthetics. These all go hand in hand to create a functional smile that's beautiful.

Dentists train in cosmetic dentistry after completing dental school. In my opinion, cosmetic dentistry is both an art and a science. I took a lot of continuing education courses on the design of a smile, because you need to be an artist. You also need to be an architect, because you're working with measurements, angulation, proportion, unity, and harmony.

Successful cosmetic dentistry reflects a balance in the composition of not only the mouth but the face as well, which includes everything from alignment to the color of the teeth. A good cosmetic dentist should have training in all of these different aspects.

Balance refers not only to the balance in the smile but also the balance between the smile and the facial features. Each patient is different. It's important to understand symmetry, because not every face is perfectly symmetrical, and we're creating a smile that needs to be in harmony with the facial symmetry or that might even improve the facial symmetry.

Continuing education is critical for the dentist to keep up to date on the whole system of full-mouth reconstruction. This includes understanding the design of the smile and all the components that come into play in terms of the shape, position, and color of the teeth. Choosing the correct shape for the teeth is an entire education in itself.

I highly recommend that dentists take courses with lab technicians, so they have an understanding of how to communicate with people who work in the laboratory. Learning the proper terminology to communicate with folks in the laboratory is critical, because a dentist may have a great idea in their mind, but, if they can't relay that to the laboratory personnel, they won't get the product they want.

Similarly, dentists must be able to communicate with their patients in a language the patients understand, so the dentist has a clear idea of what the patient wants and can also educate the patient about the problem and the process to correct it. So, whether it's with laboratory technicians or patients, good communication is crucial.

Orthodontic training has been a tremendous help in my work, because it's given me a whole foundational structure for doing minimal procedures through orthodontics. I'm able to create beautiful, healthy, harmonious smiles for my patients that are very affordable.

More than anything else, a good cosmetic dentist needs to have an understanding of the concept of unity. This means understanding that anything that you do—even in just one tooth—has an impact on the whole mouth. This is the basis of full-mouth reconstruction.

I strongly believe that having a thorough understanding of the whole masticatory system, including the temporomandibular joint, is essential for anyone to be successful at cosmetic dentistry.

Finally, a good cosmetic dentist must be passionate about what they do and really care about their patients. They look at their work as a piece of art, as a creation that changes their patient's life. That's their basic viewpoint. They're constantly striving for excellence and perfection. The successful cosmetic dentist must first be able to imagine their patient with a beautiful smile and then have the knowledge and expertise to design and execute that smile. I don't actually believe there's a specific specialization called cosmetic dentistry. It's based on imagination and artistic ability.

With every new smile I create for my patients, I feel a renewed sense of purpose along with a distinct sense of achievement, success, and the satisfaction of accomplishment. And my patients tell me I give them that same sense of accomplishment, fulfillment, and satisfaction when they go out into the world with their beautiful smiles.

In summary, a beautiful smile is important not only for aesthetic reasons but because a beautiful smile and a healthy smile are one and the same. I hope the information in this chapter has clarified how oral health and aesthetics go hand in hand.

About Mary Azadeh Afzali, DDS

Lifetime Dental
www.DoctorAfzali.com/Meet-Dr-Afzali

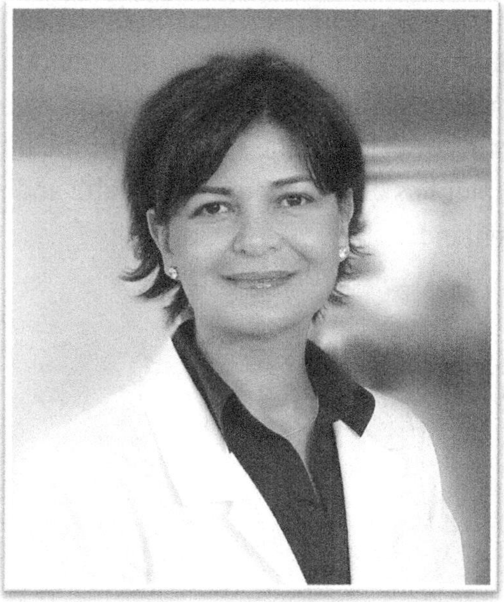

Known for her unique, holistic approach to general and cosmetic dentistry, Dr. Mary Azadeh Afzali, Founder and Clinical Director at Lifetime Dental, utilizes her nearly 30 years of clinical experience in all fields of dentistry to offer an unmatched level of care and expertise. Lifetime Dental has four offices in Southern California – in Lake Forest (Orange County), the Inland Empire, and downtown Los Angeles. Dr. Afzali has been recognized by Orange County Health & Image as a "Premier Doctor of Orange County."

Dr. Afzali addresses oral health as it relates to overall health. The focus of her post-doctoral training has been on the holistic view—looking at the big picture, the foundation and the whole body—so she can give her patients the best care. Her emphasis is on prevention and early detection of dental problems, with a special focus on orthodontics, sleep breathing disorders and correcting the bite, especially in patients who suffer from TMJ.

Dr. Afzali devotes a major portion of her practice to patient education. She believes in the human side of dentistry and medicine in general. With that in mind, she's incorporated gentle and non-toxic procedures into her four Southern California practices. Her treatments are mercury-free and metal-free. She uses aromatherapy in her practices to create a calming and pleasant experience for her patients.

Dr. Afzali achieves effective, non-surgical, soft-tissue management using laser therapy and botanical rinses to treat gum disease. She provides patients of all ages with FASTBRACES®, a patented technology that provides functional orthodontics in a fraction of the time it usually takes for regular braces. She is a certified Healthy Start Orthodontics provider and helps children and adults with sleep and breathing disorders. She was among the first group of dentists who obtained Invisalign training and certification over twenty years ago and offers her patients invisible braces as well. Her emphasis is on the art and craft of dentistry and utilizes the latest in technology available.

CROWNS... THEY'RE NOT JUST FOR ROYALTY

Smiles are the first thing we present to the world and, oftentimes, confidence and poise accompany a beautiful smile. Everyone desires a magnificent smile, and our job is to deliver that to the best of our ability.

Let me start by giving you an example of a recent patient. This patient came into my office looking for a better smile. He certainly didn't look the part of someone you would pinpoint as a cosmetic patient. He was dressed in overalls, work boots, and a tee shirt, and he had a rather large moustache that hid most of his smile. After the exam, I saw he was a tobacco chewer, and I advised him to stop that habit immediately. Together we came up with a plan of care and started the process of a full-mouth rehabilitation. This means we had to rebuild almost every tooth in his mouth.

He was thrilled with the result. In fact, he shaved the moustache and got a new haircut as well. We made an impact on this patient's everyday life, and this is exactly what state-of-the-art fillings and crowns can do.

Dental Fillings

A filling is a material that's used to replace or fill in broken or decayed areas of the tooth to restore it to its original appearance and size. There are two types of fillings commonly used: a white composite, which is made of resin and glass; and amalgam, which is made of several metals and is silver in color. A filling is used for small cracks rather than fractures. Those are usually treated with crowns, inlays, and overlays, which we'll discuss shortly.

Amalgam fillings had been the standard for years; however, in 1981, I decided to stop using them. Originally, I stopped because of the cosmetic look of the dark silver in the mouth. When a patient smiled, the tooth looked gray, or even sometimes black. It drew the eye to that area, whereas a white filling blends into the rest of the mouth.

Another negative of using the amalgams is the fact that their expansion and contraction, in response to hot and cold foods and beverages, is different than natural teeth, which can cause additional cracks in the tooth. In addition, in the early 1980s, it was discovered that some patients may have negative reactions to the mercury in the filling if it leaks out due to this expansion and contraction. This discovery was a confirmation to me to keep using the white fillings.

Even though the white filling doesn't last as long as the silver amalgam, it's a safer and more cosmetic choice. There are still some dentists that continue to use the amalgam fillings due to the fact that the technique to apply them is a bit easier than that for composite fillings, and everything in the mouth doesn't need to be so dry and isolated, which can be difficult to achieve in children. Nonetheless, I use white fillings even for baby teeth in children.

Reasons for Removing Amalgam Fillings

A valid reason for removing an amalgam filling is if there's recurrent decay happening under the filling. If this is the case, it needs to be removed and cleaned, and a determination needs to be made about how, why, and where the problem exists. Sometimes, a decay or crack can't be seen on x-rays. A patient may complain of sensitivity to hot and cold, which often accompanies a crack. In this case, the filling would need to be removed.

Although I don't remove amalgam fillings on demand, I do replace them if the patient has a concern about the cosmetic look and if there's a concern expressed by their doctor about an allergy to mercury. A recent patient had several physical challenges happening in her body, and her doctor was trying to come up with a diagnosis. Her doctor asked me to remove all the amalgam fillings and replace them with the white composite to evaluate if she was indeed allergic to mercury. Mercury toxicity exists, but it's rare. If a patient has a mouthful of silver fillings, there are procedures that medical doctors can perform to determine if an allergy or sensitivity is present.

When a patient asks for removal, I make a decision based on my assessment of the entire situation. If the filling is large, it creates a greater risk of cracking, and, if it cracks into the root, that produces an even more challenging situation.

Dental Crowns

A crown, also known as a cap, is used to cover the visible part of a tooth. In order to create such a covering, the tooth itself needs to be trimmed so the crown will fit properly. Before making a decision about a crown, other treatments must be considered and eliminated. We must determine how much tooth structure is available to use, what has been replaced by a filling, and what's the best option long-term. Once we evaluate, we can decide if a filling, an inlay, an onlay, or a crown is indicated (inlays and onlays are types of partial crowns, and we'll discuss them later).

Sometimes that determination is made after we address the crack and decay. I'd much rather be conservative than aggressive and keep as much natural tooth structure as possible.

There are many different types of crowns and many materials used in making them. For the front teeth, a white material was developed in the 1980s that's made of acrylic. It isn't very strong and doesn't work well long-term; however, this material is still used in temporary crowns today.

The next development was porcelain fused to a metal crown. Porcelain itself isn't a strong material, so it was necessary to bind it to an underlying metal. This type of crown provides strength and a nice cosmetic appearance. The porcelain-over-metal crown was a standard for many years; however, it does present a disadvantage. The metal can block light and create an opaque and chalky look under the porcelain, thereby eliminating the bright and translucent light we see in a natural tooth. This crown is still widely used, especially for bridge work.

The industry is now migrating to an E-MAX crown or an all-white crown. This is stronger and much more durable than porcelain and acrylic crowns. They're cosmetically gorgeous as well. The E-MAX has become the new standard for front teeth.

An alternative option is veneers and crowns made of feldspathic material, which are drop-dead gorgeous! They look completely natural. No one would ever question if these are natural teeth. I use them more for front teeth, where cosmetics is most important, and mostly for veneers. I use a lab in Hollywood to help create these WOW! smiles.

Another type of crown is a zirconia crown, which is very durable and probably the strongest on the market aside from metal crowns. The zirconia is much prettier than the older metal crowns. It doesn't transfer light very well; however, the zirconia anterior crown is more translucent and more eye pleasing than other metal-based crowns.

Gold crowns were a standard in years past and are sometimes still an option. A yellow-gold crown is a conservative approach, because it doesn't require trimming too much of the tooth structure. In addition, the expansion and contraction of a gold crown is very similar to that of a natural tooth.

In addition to gold crowns, there are nonprecious metal crowns with the appearance of shiny nickel. They're a little less costly but aren't used very often in today's dentistry. They're durable but not as cosmetically pleasing.

Choosing the Right Crown

When a patient comes for a consultation, the dentist should explain all the options and what they recommend and why. I want my patients to understand exactly what I'm going to do and why I'm doing it.

If we strictly focus on cosmetics, a feldspathic crown is an excellent option. The material is fantastic for the veneer of a three-quarter crown applied to the front teeth. The bite and natural teeth' structure are maintained, so the focus remains on the cosmetic.

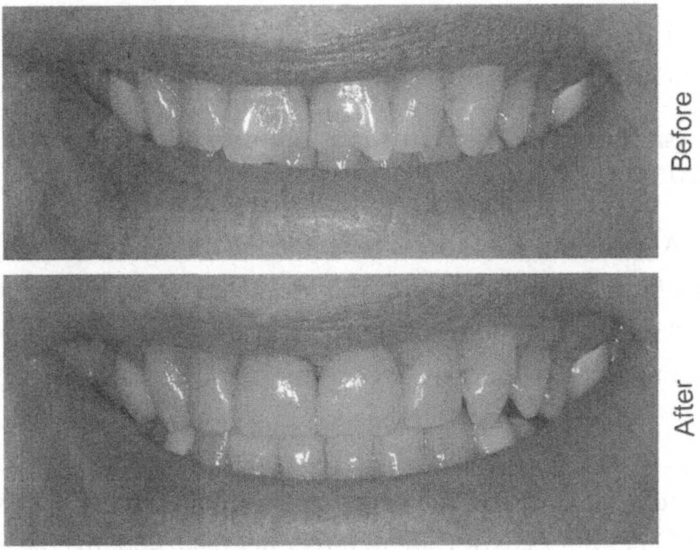

Before and after placing crowns

If the focus is on something very durable and cosmetics are secondary (such as with the back teeth), my choice would be a gold or silver crown—or, if a patient doesn't want metal, a zirconia crown. If the tooth indicated is in between the front and back, I recommend an E-MAX crown, because it offers more strength than the feldspathic but not as much as a zirconia.

Inlays or Onlays

At times, a filling isn't sufficient to repair a cracked or decayed tooth, and a crown isn't indicated. In these cases, a dentist may suggest an inlay or an onlay. An inlay is placed on top of the surface of the tooth but doesn't cover the cusps; in contrast, an onlay covers the entire surface of the tooth. Both are made of porcelain material and restore a tooth to its natural appearance and size. Inlays and onlays offer the conservative approach of a filling with the strength and cosmetic advantages of a crown.

Case Study: Restoring a Smile and Changing a Life

A patient in her forties came into the office after driving two hours to meet with us. She presented with headaches, acid reflux, sleep apnea, and was a grinder, meaning she'd ground her teeth down to one-third of their natural size. As a result, she was embarrassed to smile and had the appearance of a much older woman. She expressed that she'd been to several dentists before coming to my office. I told her my Plan of Care to repair her teeth and give her a beautiful smile. She conveyed that she felt totally disabled by the teeth she had. She said her teeth not only affected her personal life but her business relationships as well, because she rarely smiled and, therefore, she came off to others as angry.

My Plan of Care included different materials for different areas of her mouth—some materials for strength, because of the grinding, and some for cosmetics. First, we needed to realign her TMJ or jaw joint, which was done with splint therapy. Her treatment plan took longer than a usual case due to this fact. We also treated her sleep apnea right away.

She was absolutely thrilled with the end result. Not only did she look like a model, but she was headache-free! On the day of final treatment, we handed her a mirror. She burst into tears and started hugging us. She told us that we'd changed her life and said, "Now I can be who God wanted me to be." This statement was powerful to hear and reminded us why we do what we do every day.

Creating Crowns

Most crowns, as well as inlays and onlays, are manufactured in an off-site dental lab. It's imperative to use a high-quality lab to assure that the color matching and functional factors are state-of-the-art. The patient will have two separate appointments with their dentist—one for impressions and the other for installing the crown. The time period between appointments can be two to three weeks depending on the speed of the lab.

During the first appointment, the dentist will take impressions of the patient's mouth and will make a temporary or transitional crown to put over the tooth. That will be worn until the second appointment, when the permanent crown is placed.

In recent years, it's become possible to create crowns, inlays, and onlays inside the dental office during a single appointment. This is accomplished by using an intraoral scanner to make a digital impression and a CEREC machine to create the crown, inlay, or onlay. The scanner avoids the need for impression materials to be used inside the patient's mouth. This is a tremendous advantage for those patients with a strong gag reflex.

The CEREC can create crowns, inlays, and onlays in many different materials including acrylic, E-MAX, zirconia, etc. All of this can be accomplished in one appointment within 90 minutes.

Many dentists still prefer to use a lab to create a crown, but I find there are a number of benefits to using a CEREC machine. First, the machine offers the same degree of cosmetic quality as an off-site lab, because the filling or crown can be perfectly matched to the tooth color. Second, the material used is much stronger than the composite material, and it's processed differently. The wear factor is very similar to a natural tooth.

Another positive of the one-day crown is if the patient needs to be sedated. Using the CEREC will eliminate the need for a second appointment of sedation. This is a big positive for those patients who are uncomfortable with anesthesia.

Some patients struggle to find time in their schedules to get to the dental office, so opting for the one-day crown eliminates the need to find two openings in their already full calendars.

In my office, I do about 95% digital scanning, and around 90% of my inlays and onlays are done in-house in one day. I continue to use the lab for cosmetic work.

How Durable Are Crowns?

This question comes up quite often with my patients, and I tell them I've never seen a crown that didn't last into the double digits in terms of years. I've had patients who had crowns installed in the 1980s that are still perfect. I give a warranty on my crowns with a stipulation that the patient does their part and adheres to the instructions on how to maintain the crown. This includes proper hygiene, coming into the office for check-ups four times a year, and doing nothing that will abuse the crown.

FAQs

How Much Will a Crown Cost?

The cost of a crown can vary based on the dentist's expertise, geographic location, and lab charges for labor and materials, just to name a few. Costs can range from $900-$3,000. I try and price my crowns between $950-$1,500 depending on the type of crown used. I try and ensure an affordable crown while still maintaining a high quality of functionality and beauty.

Is It Going to Hurt?

The process of installing a crown, inlay, or onlay involves the use of local anesthesia to ensure patients are comfortable throughout the procedure. So, aside from the small pinch with the injection, the process is painless.

What Will It Look Like?

The crown should look as close as possible to a natural tooth. In some cases, such as when a tooth is missing or needs to be reshaped, it can be hard for a patient to imagine how the new crown will look. Different dentists have different methods to solve that. I can share what I do.

To make sure patients are able to visualize how they'll look, we offer what's called a mock-up. I have everything waxed up ahead of the patient's appointment. When the patient arrives, we place the mock-up in their mouth so they're able to actually see what they'll look like and not just view it on a computer screen.

We also offer before-and-after photos to help the patient see the tooth or teeth before treatment, and why we propose the changes that are in our Plan of Care. We use an intraoral camera to take a photo of the patient's tooth before we do any work and put the picture on the computer for the patient to see. We then begin to trim the tooth and remove what's needed for the crown to fit properly. We restore the tooth by installing the filling, onlay, or crown and take a second picture. The patient is always amazed seeing the side-by-side photos.

There are many advances in the dental field that offer diverse choices for the patient when it comes to fillings and crowns. I hope I was able to explain all the options available to assist you in making the right choice for you.

Keep smiling.

About Ricardo Zambito, DDS

Zambito Family Dentistry
www.ZambitoDentistry.com

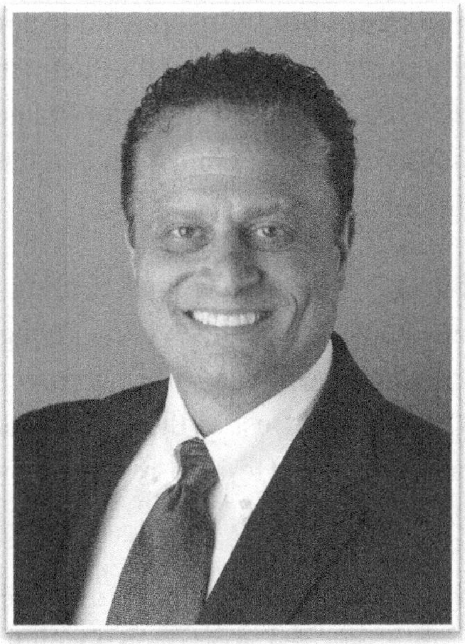

In 1980, Dr. Ricardo Zambito obtained a Doctor of Dental Surgery degree from the West Virginia University School of Dentistry. He has focused his dental practice on family dentistry with an emphasis on high-tech solutions for dental problems. He describes his practice with the phrase, "State of the art with a family heart."

Dr. Zambito ("Dr. Z", as his patients call him) has specialized training in cosmetics and facial aesthetics as well as implant dentistry. He has numerous certifications including laser dentistry, CAD/CAM systems, and implantology as well as therapeutic Botox and facial aesthetics. This background allows him to accomplish a complete transformation in his patients' appearance while assisting them to achieve their dental health goals.

Dr. Zambito shares his philosophy and expertise in lectures and demonstrations presented to dentists across the nation, and he's the founder of Integrity Practice Management. He enjoys continuing education and has completed thousands of hours of courses.

Dr. Zambito is also on staff at Wheeling Hospital, is the acting consultant dentist for several nursing homes, and was the recipient of the West Virginia Governor Service Award in 2019 and the "Best of the Ohio Valley Readers' Choice" award in 2019. He also received the American Top Dentist Award for 2020.

Among the professional societies of which Dr. Zambito is a member, are the American Dental Association (ADA), Academy of General Dentistry (AGD), American College of Dentists (ACD), and the West Virginia Dental Association (WVDA). He has had fellowships with the American Academy of Facial Esthetics (AAFE) and Midwest Implant Institute (MII).

Dr. Zambito's pride and joy are his wife of 43 years, Cheryl, and their three children and six grandchildren.

Brighten Your Smile with Teeth Whitening

One of the first things that people notice about us is our smile. Our smile conveys a tremendous amount of information about who we are, and it also influences how people respond to us. A beautiful smile draws people to us and makes them feel welcome. A dazzling white smile isn't only beautiful in itself, but it lets people know that we care about ourselves and our appearance.

In our current culture, people are more aware of their smile and of the brightness of their teeth. Everyone wants to have that Hollywood smile—those perfectly white, straight teeth. There's a lot of social pressure to have cosmetically beautiful teeth, and this means white teeth.

Here's an example of how whitening the teeth can transform an individual's life. A gentleman in his mid-30s came into our office. He was friendly, but he didn't smile, so we assumed he was self-conscious about his teeth. Indeed, he came to us because he wanted to have them whitened.

The day we did the whitening procedure, he hung out for a little while afterwards and chatted with us. All the while, he was smiling. He kept taking pictures with his phone of himself smiling. Gazing at the photos made him smile even more. It was like his whole personality had been transformed. He went from a guy who was almost melancholy to engaging with us and laughing. His whole attitude changed that day.

Another psychological and health advantage to whitening the teeth is that some patients, after they've had whitening done, start paying more attention to other dental issues and are motivated to address those.

Teeth whitening has become very popular over the last couple of decades, and a variety of whitening products and processes are available—both for use in the dentist's office and at home. I'm going to talk about professional teeth whitening as well as teeth-whitening kits that can be purchased over-the-counter—including the disadvantages of the latter. But first, let's learn what causes tooth discoloration in the first place.

Causes of Tooth Discoloration

The most common cause of tooth staining is the food and drinks that we consume—in particular, coffee and tea. The popularity of Starbucks and similar places has shown us that many people are consuming these specialty coffee drinks on a regular basis.

Beets, in particular, and dark, leafy greens can also discolor teeth, and we advise that people don't eat beets after their teeth have been whitened. Red wine is another contributor to tooth staining.

Of course, the use of tobacco products has long been known to be a main cause of tooth discoloration. Also, there are a number of medications that can discolor teeth, such as allergy medicines that contain antihistamines. Many patients take maintenance medications such as antipsychotic drugs and medications to treat blood pressure, and these also can change the color of the teeth.

Who Typically Seeks Out Teeth Whitening and Why

The typical age range of people seeking teeth whitening used to be folks in their 30s, 40s, and 50s, but now even teenagers are coming to dentists seeking this treatment, because they want to look like the stars they see on social media. Also, members of our older population are starting to show interest in whitening their teeth. Maybe they're thinking of getting back into the dating scene and are therefore more concerned about aesthetics, or they want that boost of self-esteem that a brighter smile provides.

Life events—in particular, weddings, proms, graduations, or looking for a job or wanting to change jobs—are another major reason that people have their teeth whitened. Spring is often when dentists have the most business from people seeking teeth whitening in preparation for a wedding or graduation.

Teeth Whitening Treatments—Professional and Over-the-Counter

In my 17 years of practice, I've seen the options for teeth whitening change and expand to include a number of different methods. The traditional professional methods are in-office treatments and at-home treatments, both of which are prescribed by and managed by a dentist. There's also an array of over-the-counter teeth-whitening products that people can purchase in their grocery store or pharmacy as well as products that can be ordered online. In addition, places like beauty salons and spas sometimes offer teeth whitening as one of their services. The availability of these products is an indicator of the perceived importance of having white teeth among a growing number of the general public.

I strongly recommend professional teeth whitening, and I'll explain why. First of all, it's critical to have a dental exam and cleaning before beginning any type of whitening procedure. If the patient chooses an in-office whitening treatment, this is completed in one appointment.

The other option is to whiten their teeth at home using trays that are worn for a certain period of time. In the in-office method, we isolate the teeth from the surrounding tissue, which means we can use higher levels of peroxide to whiten them. The whitening process is carried out under careful supervision based on professional standards and techniques.

If the patient opts to do the whitening at home, we design trays that are customized for each patient, and a peroxide gel is used as the whitening agent. Even though this is done at home, the dentist is still overseeing the whitening process. We monitor the patient to make sure the appropriate and desired shade is being reached and the patient is complying with our instructions. Of course, in-office treatment allows us to achieve better results in terms of getting a particular shade of whiteness. We can use laser light to enhance the whitening process as well.

The main difference between in-office treatment and at-home treatment is the time frame for results—an hour or so in the office, in which two or three whitening sessions are completed, versus up to two weeks to achieve the same degree of whitening at home with one, 15- to 30-minute session a day.

Concerns About Over-the-Counter Whitening Products

Although whitening products purchased online or over-the counter do work, we have concerns about them being overused or improperly used, which can damage the teeth and the gum tissue if not used properly or if used too frequently. Also, the trays used in commercial teeth-whitening systems aren't customized to the individual's mouth like the trays that dentists use. In the office, we scan or take impressions of that patient's mouth, and we make trays to fit their mouth and their teeth. In this way, we're able to control where the whitening gel goes. With a commercial product that has a one-size-fits-all tray, the gel may get on the gums as well as the teeth, because there's not as much control of where the gel goes. Much better results are achieved using a customized tray that a dentist creates. Also, there aren't the concerns about burning of the gums or the lips, which can happen when using a tray that isn't customized to the person's mouth.

The agents used in whitening can cause additional damage to the gum tissue if it's inflamed, if disease or tooth decay is present, or if there are other problems going on in the mouth. I've had countless instances of patients who've come into my office after they've whitened their teeth at home with an over-the-counter product and had unexpected side effects. The home whitening process caused their teeth to become sensitive or brought to light some other problem that they hadn't had evaluated by a dentist.

Although whitening is a very safe procedure if carried out by a dentist, over-the-counter whitening systems contain high concentrations of peroxide, which can be harmful if used too frequently or improperly, as previously mentioned. In the same way, some toothpastes and homemade teeth-whitening products like the combination of baking soda and peroxide can damage tooth enamel.

The loss of enamel causes tooth sensitivity. There's a chemical additive in teeth-whitening products that can cause this, and whitening products that contain abrasives can physically remove the enamel structure from the teeth. Sensitivity results when there's no longer a sufficient layer of enamel to protect the tooth from pain caused by exposure to cold, heat, and certain foods.

Charcoal is another popular method that people are using to whiten their teeth. While all of the methods I mentioned do work and will remove surface staining from the teeth, the concern is that, over time, the abrasiveness of these products thins the enamel and causes damage to the gum tissue.

Also, when the enamel thins, the yellow dentin beneath the enamel starts to show through and gives the teeth a yellow hue—which can't be remedied. I've had patients come into my office and tell me, "I've been whitening, whitening, whitening for so long, but it seems like my teeth are getting darker." Well, the teeth aren't getting darker. What's happening is the yellow dentin layer under the enamel is starting to show through.

The Advantages of Having a Dental Professional Whiten Your Teeth

So, it's clear that without an understanding of the tooth structure and the effects of certain products on the teeth—which are things a dental professional knows—it might not only be disappointing but dangerous to attempt teeth whitening on your own at home.

Teeth whitening is safe if done by a professional. The main complaints that dentists hear have to do with unrealistic patient expectations rather than problems with the treatment itself. If gums or teeth have problems, these can be exacerbated by the application of peroxide. For example, 80% of people have gum problems (and many are unaware of them), so these may be worsened by exposing the gums to peroxide. Also, plaque and tartar won't whiten, so a thorough cleaning as well as repairing any cavities should be addressed first. In our office, we always clean the patient's teeth prior to whitening them even if the patient has had their teeth cleaned just a few months previously.

Another consideration is that restorations like veneers and crowns don't respond to the whitening process, and this can lead to disappointing results. The fact that restorations aren't affected by whitening agents is another reason to have a dental professional do it. They can whiten the teeth first and match subsequent restorations to that shade.

In-office Whitening Treatments

During my years of practice, I've worked with three or four different whitening systems—Zoom and Opalescence among them. I've had about the same success with the various products, because I've discovered the technique is more important than the product. For example, KöR Whitening is a detailed and extensive procedure, but most of the other products I've used accomplish the same degree of whitening.

The most popular professional whitening system right now is the Opalescence prefilled trays. They're available in concentrations of 6%, 10%, and 30% hydrogen peroxide. The degree of concentration we choose depends on how long we leave the tray in the patient's mouth. With over-the counter products, there's no rhyme or reason for how long the patient uses them based on the concentration.

For some whitening systems, it's recommended that in-home trays remain in the patient's mouth overnight. The amount of peroxide in those trays is 15%. In our office, we use concentrations up to 35%, which demonstrates the difference in the concentration that we're comfortable using in the office versus at home. Sad to say, I've seen products available for purchase online that have these high concentrations of peroxide. It's very concerning that the average consumer is using these products at home without supervision.

Professional tooth whitening lasts two or three years, depending on the patient's diet, whether they continue to drink coffee or tea, and whether they continue to smoke, etc. All of these habits will result in the teeth becoming stained again and losing brilliance. The extent to which patients change the habits that cause teeth staining determines, to a large part, when the teeth will need to be whitened again.

The normal protocol in our office is that we can always whiten the teeth again after a year or so. Because we make customized trays for patients who get in-office whitening, they don't necessarily have to have the subsequent treatment done in the office. When they start to see some discoloration reappearing, we provide them with the whitening gel, which they use in the tray for a few days. In this way, the teeth can usually be whitened to their previous brightness.

Reasons Why Tooth Whitening May Not Be Recommended

If a patient already has issues with tooth sensitivity, we don't recommend whitening unless we're able to correct the tooth sensitivity. Also, there are some patients that aren't willing or committed to changing their habits for a couple of weeks during the whitening process. For example, if they smoke or drink red wine—and they aren't able to stop smoking or consuming red wine for those two weeks—we don't recommend whitening, because it just won't be effective.

In addition, there are certain medical conditions that may influence whether teeth whitening is a good idea. For example, we don't recommend whitening for people undergoing chemotherapy or radiation therapy.

There's no problem with pregnant women having their teeth whitened, but we advise that this be done in-office so we can control the process and there's no chance of any of the product being ingested.

Insurance doesn't cover tooth whitening, because it's considered cosmetic. The one exception might be a procedure called internal bleaching, which is mostly done as a result of trauma to a tooth or because of congenital or tetracycline staining. These cases require much more extensive work and bleaching.

The cost of in-office tooth whitening is usually between \$300 to \$400. I've seen it be more than that, and I've seen it be less with that, particularly when dental offices have to compete with salons or other non-dental professionals that offer whitening. Over the years, I've tried to maintain an affordable price for in-office whitening and communicate to my patients the importance and the benefits of doing in-office whitening versus having a nonprofessional do it or doing it at home with over-the-counter whitening products or products purchased online.

About Nekia Staley-Neither, DDS

Special Care Dentistry
www.MySpecialDentist.com

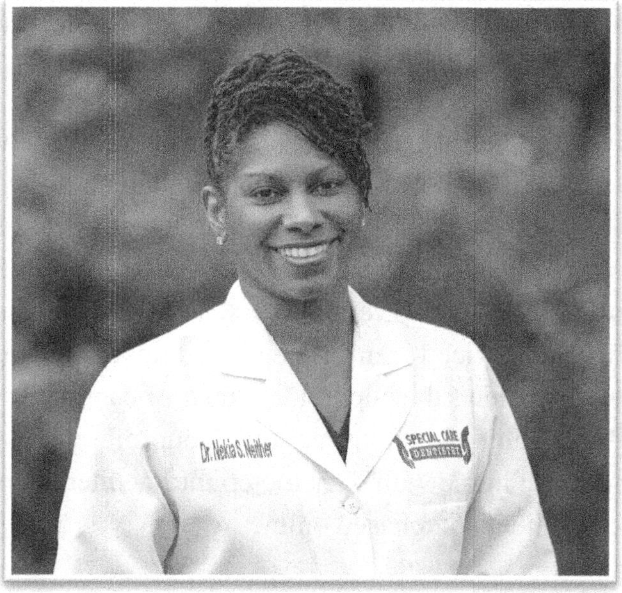

Dr. Nekia Staley-Neither is native Washingtonian. She grew up with a love for caring for others with special interest in medicine. She matriculated at Spelman College in Atlanta, Georgia as a pre-med Biology major. After choosing to pursue a career in dentistry she attended and graduated from Howard University College of Dentistry with a degree in Doctor of Dental Surgery.

Dr. Staley-Neither is a dedicated wife and mother of four beautiful daughters and two sons. She is an active member of Mt. Ennon Baptist Church. Dr. Neither also, volunteers as the Artistic Director of Standing Ovations Dance Academy in District Heights, Maryland.

Enhancing Dr. Staley-Neither's commitment to providing care to person of all background she is a Decod Fellow at the University of Washington at Seattle where she has and continues to train to treat and accommodate mentally and physically challenged person. Dr. Neither has been involved with the special needs community since her elementary years. Volunteering at the Hospital for sick children and various shelters in Atlanta where she completed her undergraduate studies.

Dr. Staley-Neither is a member of the American Dental Association and National Dental Association. She is the founder and president of Special Care For Special Needs Dentistry, a non-profit organization established to serve special needs patients and their caregivers. You can also find Dr. Staley-Neither participating, sponsoring, and serving in various health fairs, dental fairs and other community service projects in the Washington Metropolitan Area. Annually Dr. Staley-Neither host and sponsors a community day at one of her practice location giving away free dentistry for the community at large. She is a caring and committed professional who is dedicated to her patient's overall health.

THE FOUNDATION OF A GREAT SMILE

All patients should understand the relationship between their teeth and gums by thinking of a photograph in a frame. The teeth are the center point of a photo while the gums provide the support. If the framework is out of line or damaged, then the photo in the center will not appear as beautiful as it would if the border were in perfect working order and alignment.

ISSUES WITH GUMS AND TEETH

All patients, even those not concerned with cosmetic dentistry, should brush and floss their teeth and gums daily to prevent gum and tooth diseases. In addition to maintaining good oral hygiene, patients should also receive a dental checkup and cleaning every six months. For patients interested in cosmetic dentistry, good oral hygiene and routine dental visits are crucial. With cosmetic dentistry, the first step is to determine whether or not the gums are healthy. If your gums look red, swollen, inflamed, and bleeding, those are warning signs of an infection. If your gums are infected, then your dentist has to take care of that issue before proceeding to cosmetic dentistry. Again, think of the gums and the underlying bone as the foundation for your teeth. It is critical to make sure that supporting base is solid first, and then the dentist can build on that strong framework to achieve the goal of making your teeth and smile as esthetically beautiful as possible.

Depending on the nature of the inflammation or infection, there are surgical and non-surgical treatments that may be used to correct the problem.

Besides the physical appearance of the gums, it is also important to look at the height of your teeth in relation to your gums – the proportion between your gums and the teeth. If your teeth appear short, this may be because gum tissue is covering part of the bottom portion of the teeth so that they are not visible. This can happen in young adults – men and women in their teens, twenties, or thirties – if their gums have not migrated to their proper final location. The gums have stopped short of settling into their appropriate location, and this can leave part of your adult teeth hidden under your gums.

Your teeth may naturally appear a little bit "short" when you are a child and teenager, but by the time you are a full-grown adult, your gums should have finished migrating to their appropriate position in your mouth. But many times – especially in the esthetic zone – the gums stop migrating too soon, which can give you short-looking teeth.

As you age, the opposite problem can occur – your teeth may appear unnaturally long. That is where the expression "long in the tooth" comes from – which means a person looks old. If your gums have migrated past the point where they are supposed to be, it is commonly referred to as receding gums.

Receding gums cause the "long in the tooth" appearance. Gum recession may occur gradually or rapidly. Many people that show a lot of teeth when the smile, laugh, or speak may consciously or subconsciously try to hide this by covering their mouth with their hand or by intentionally not lifting their upper lip.

In these clinical situations, teeth looking too short or teeth that appear too long, there are dental procedures that can be used to put your gum tissue in its normal, proper location in order to fix the problem.

Gums and Cosmetic Dentistry

You know, patients do not usually come to see a dentist and say, "Can you check out my gums?" No, they come to my office and want to know, "Can you make my teeth look nicer?" That is all right – I do not expect the patient to be an expert on gum disease and gum location and to know, without being educated about it, that the right thing to do is secure the foundation of your teeth – the gums – before trying to do any work on their teeth appearance.

Dentists have an ethical obligation to inform you about your complete oral health. A good dentist should be honest enough to inform you: "Look, there is no point in you investing your time and hard-earned money in, say, tooth whitening, if you have gum disease that, untreated, could make you lose those nice, white teeth. So first, let us take care of any gum disease issues, and then we can talk about cosmetic procedures". That is the dentist's job as a medical professional, to take the time to educate you, the patient, so that you can make intelligently informed choices.

And when dentists and their staff do that – make a concerted effort to educate patients so that they understand basic concepts to include gum disease and recession – then the patient not only gets what they really want but also what they need to achieve a great-looking smile.

Dentists should not be talking about merely the appearance of individual teeth, but about the total look of your smile, which includes the appearance of your gums in relation to the lips and face. Fortunately, more and more dentists are taking a holistic approach, discussing how your overall health affects the health of your teeth and gums – not their appearance.

In my professional opinion, all cosmetic dental procedures should begin with an evaluation and appropriate treatment of your gums before treating the teeth. The bottom line is that cosmetic procedures such as veneers or orthodontic treatments should not be undertaken unless your gums and supporting bone are already healthy or after successful gum treatments.

Cosmetic Gum Treatments - Correcting the "Short Teeth" Look

In addition to treating gum disease, I also perform cosmetic gum procedures. One of the most common cosmetic treatments for gums is correcting the condition where a patient's gum tissue is cover too much of the bottom portion of his or her teeth, giving the appearance of having short or tiny-looking teeth.

Your teeth come out of the bone of your skull – specifically, your jaw bone. When you are a small child you have "baby" teeth, and then your adult teeth follow those teeth. This occurs in two phases: active and passive. The active eruption phase is the teeth coming out of the bone, the part we are all familiar with, your adult teeth coming in to replace your lost "baby teeth".

But there is also a passive eruption phase that is the gum tissue migrating – moving – into its final, mature location around the neck of each tooth.

When that passive phase occurs correctly, the tooth is properly exposed above your gum line, and everything looks how it is supposed to. However, when the gum tissue does not settle down properly around the neck of the tooth, an excessive amount of gum tissue is covering part of the enamel of your teeth, making them appear short. This tends to make adults, when they smile or speak, look like they have child-sized teeth.

In layman's terms, this condition is often referred to as having a "gummy smile" which can be corrected with a simple procedure called esthetic crown lengthening. That phrase sounds like a mouthful, I know, but it is really a fairly simple procedure, designed to make sure the teeth appear to be properly proportioned in relation to the gums.

The periodontist first examines the teeth and takes all the necessary measurements. The front six to ten teeth, depending on how wide the patient can smile, are anesthetized. The procedure begins with a gingivectomy, in which the periodontist removes a precise number of millimeters of gum tissue on each tooth involved, based on the measurements taken previously. Then, the periodontist re-contours the bone, creating the ideal relationship of bone to gum and tooth. Esthetic crown lengthening is a common procedure performed before veneers and crowns are fabricated and during, or at the conclusion of, orthodontics, i.e., braces.

I recommend that patients find a board-certified periodontist who is always up to date on cutting-edge dental technology. Having a skilled dental professional who utilizes the latest surgical techniques makes all the difference in the world as far as having the absolute best clinical outcome and overall patient experience with minimal discomfort. Newer, less-invasive dental procedures continue to be target of the most innovations in periodontics.

Highly skilled periodontists (and dentists) are also gentle with their approaches. They can do extensive dental work on your teeth and gums without leaving you in a lot of pain when the anesthetic wears off. In the case of esthetic crown lengthening, the patient usually leaves the periodontist's office with a few stitches that will dissolve over the next couple of weeks. Then the patient will come back a few weeks later so that the periodontist can take a look and make sure that the gums have healed properly, and that the patient has gotten the look they want for their smile.

One of the greatest benefits of the esthetic crown lengthening procedure is that it is something a periodontist can do in about an hour and then the patient can see instantaneous results.

The cost for a cosmetic treatment like this, depending mostly on how many teeth are involved, usually runs from two to three thousand dollars. That is a fair price considering orthodontic treatment can cost double to move teeth. There is always the question of whether insurance will cover this procedure. However, every plan, and every insurance company, is different. Typically, dental insurance, like medical insurance, does not cover cosmetic procedures. If a patient has to cover the majority of the costs themselves, most dental offices will offer them a number of payment options to lessen the financial burden.

Cosmetic Gum Treatments - Correcting Gum Recession

Unlike excessive gums, gum recession is when the teeth appear longer than they ideally should be, usually as a result of periodontitis, although there can be other causes, such as a patient having thin gum tissue. The quality and quantity of the gum tissue plays a vital role in preventing or exacerbating gum recession. The position of your teeth in relation to your jawbone can cause the “long in the tooth” look, too.

In some cases, this condition can be caused by hard tooth brushing over a period of years, especially with hard or firm bristle toothbrushes. Some patients, who brush their teeth and gums too aggressively, inadvertently cause the gum tissue to move down the tooth and expose the roots. This is one of the reasons it is always recommended for patients to utilize soft bristled toothbrushes since medium and hard bristled toothbrushes can accelerate gum recession. Basically, there are a number of things that, as people naturally age, can cause gum recession and elongated teeth.

One contributing factor for gum recession is being in orthodontics or having a history of orthodontic treatment. Teeth usually erupt where the bone is the thickest. Often, the spot where the bone is the thickest is not the precise spot where the teeth need to be in order to be perfectly aligned.

As the orthodontist attempts to align the teeth and put them into the correct location, he or she begins moving the teeth outward towards the lips and cheeks. For many patients, the bone and gum tissue is significantly thinner towards the lips and cheeks. In any event, it is not uncommon for patients who have had braces to start experiencing gum recession, even though they do not actually have any active gum disease.

I am very much in favor of using a multi-disciplinary approach to cosmetic dentistry, where general dentistry practitioners, along with appropriate specialists, all work together to evaluate patients and design the best possible plan for each individual.

Let me illustrate how that works in practice. For example, sometimes with patients who receive orthodontics treatment, the orthodontist will have a periodontist perform preventive gum grafting procedures if the patient has noticeably thin gum tissue or the tissue has already receded. Gum grafting prior to or during orthodontic treatment can prevent gum recession problems from occurring in the future.

Gum Disease Conditions That Require Treatment

There are two basic types of gum disease – gingivitis and periodontitis. Gingivitis shows up as inflamed, irritated, or bleeding gums. The more serious kind of gum disease is periodontitis, where you have actually had some bone loss around your teeth. Periodontitis can be mild, moderate, or severe and lead to tooth loss.

Periodontal disease is very common. The American Academy of Periodontology states that one out of two adults over the age of thirty have some form of periodontitis. Some patients are born with a genetic predisposition to develop periodontal disease. Others may develop it because of poor oral hygiene, having comorbid systemic diseases, and/or because they use tobacco products. If you have been going to your dentist regularly for several years and receiving adequate treatment all along, then there is a good chance that you have been able to catch early on any gum disease that may have developed, and successfully treat it with non-surgical procedures. In that case, if you start thinking about some cosmetic dental work that you may want to have done, then you are probably in a position to go right ahead with getting cosmetic dental work after discussing treatment options with your dentist and deciding on a treatment option.

On the other hand, with a new patient, especially one who has not been receiving regular dental care for a number of years, there is a good chance that the dentist will need to address some gum disease problems before being in a position to do any cosmetic work the patient wants.

Performing a complete assessment of the condition of a patient's gums, which includes full mouth probe depths and radiographs, allows a periodontist to determine whether they have gingivitis or periodontitis. If the patient has gingivitis, that can usually be corrected with non-surgical treatment, and then he or she can go ahead with orthodontic or other cosmetic treatment after a couple of months.

With periodontitis, if there is only mild bone loss, then the nonsurgical procedure of choice is scaling and root planning, what patients may know as "deep cleaning". It is a little more than your typical cleaning when you go to the dentist. The main difference is that the dentist will give you a local anesthetic for the deep cleaning on those teeth that have mild periodontal disease.

A deep cleaning treatment usually takes about two, two-hour appointments that allow adequate time for dental anesthesia and for the hygienists to do a thorough job. In addition to removing bacteria with the cleaning, the entire dental team will spend a great deal of time educating the patient, so that they can change their dental care habits and hopefully avoid ever getting more severe forms of periodontitis. This is crucial to changing the dental habits of patient and needs to be reinforced at future appointments.

I tell patients all the time that every single tooth could have a completely different periodontal diagnosis. You might have a completely healthy tooth, next to a tooth with gingivitis, next to a tooth with severe periodontitis. And in all of those situations, the treatment is different.

However, if you have moderate to severe periodontitis that typically requires a surgical procedure, you will probably be treated then maintained for a period of six to twelve months depending on the specific surgery and course of treatment. It is important to take care of periodontitis, because otherwise – if you do not get the gums and bone around your teeth healthy – then whatever cosmetic treatment you receive may be a waste of your time and money.

I always try to make sure patients do understand this: It is crucial to first make sure the supporting foundation is in good shape before investing money in cosmetic procedures to give you that really beautiful smile. Again, it may be helpful to recall the analogy of a photo and a frame. Your "photo" (teeth) is never going to look like you want it to if the picture "frame" (gums) is seriously damaged.

Risks of Untreated Gum Recession

It is important to understand what a potentially serious problem gum recession is if left untreated. If you have gum recession and do not get the proper treatment for it, you are at a significantly increased risk for tooth sensitivity, root cavities, and overall tooth loss.

The greater the amount of recession, the more likely you are to ultimately lose a tooth – or multiple teeth. The exposure of the root surface of a tooth leaves you much more vulnerable to getting root cavities – cavities that occur on the bottom part of the exposed tooth, above the gum line.

Root cavities are particularly dangerous, as compared to a cavity in the body or top portion of a tooth, because the cavity is eating away the structure that holds the tooth in place in your jaw, and that is why tooth loss is a real possibility.

As we age, many adults develop systemic diseases that require medications. Unfortunately, one of the many side effects of these medications is decreasing the amount of saliva creating a condition called dry mouth. Dry mouth, while annoying to the patient, can be detrimental to the teeth – especially if the teeth have experienced gingival recession increasing the chance of root cavities.

Root cavities are different than regular cavities. Most people are probably familiar with the term "enamel", which is the protective coating that usually covers each of your teeth. Enamel is pretty resistant to cavities, although of course, patients with poor oral hygiene and poor diet can get cavities through your tooth enamel.

The main reason root cavities differ from cavities in the in the enamel is the gum recession has exposed a different part of the tooth – the cementum-covered root, a part of the tooth that is not normally exposed. What is different about the root is that there is no protective enamel covering on the root part of your teeth. The enamel is designed to protect the upper, outer portion of your teeth, and the gum tissue is supposed to protect the root of the tooth. But if your gums recede, then that protection for the root of your tooth is not there. Once you start to acquire a root cavity, the cavity gets worse much quicker, the damage advances more rapidly. After a very short period of time, the damage can quickly reach the point where there is nothing your dentist can do to save the tooth, and it has to be removed.

I cannot stress enough that if you have gum recession, you need to get it treated as soon as possible. Once you lose an adult tooth, it is not coming back. This is why it is critical for you to visit a dentist every six months. The main early warning sign of gum disease is bleeding of the gums. But one thing I should mention is that people who use tobacco products may not show that early warning sign. That is because tobacco products constrict your blood vessels, which makes you less prone to bleeding. That is another reason I tell my patients that everyone should be evaluated at a dental office twice a year.

Treatment for Gum Recession with Periodontal Plastic Surgery

The traditional way to treat gum recession is by using time-tested gingival grafting technique that has been around for many years. This treatment involves harvesting a free-gingival graft or the underlying connective tissue from the patient's palate, to use as donor tissue, which is then sutured or stitched into place in the area of the gum where there is gum recession. The patient's natural gum tissue that is below the recession is stitched up over the top of the grafted area.

The advantage of this technique is that the dentist is using the patient's own tissue for the procedure, transplanting the patient's gum tissue from one location to another.

But the disadvantage is that there is usually multiple teeth requiring treatment, and there is only so much tissue available from the palate that can be transplanted. So it is difficult, if not impossible, to get enough tissue to completely take care of everything. Furthermore, harvesting tissue from the palate causes discomfort for the patient, which is something periodontists really try to avoid nowadays.

If you have several teeth requiring treatment for gum recession, then this traditional gum grafting approach is neither realistic nor practical. There is a limited amount of tissue to work with, plus, it would take multiple visits and procedures over several months or years, something most patients are unwilling to do.

Because of the limitations with using the traditional gum grafting procedure, the mid-1990s brought about a new approach in the treatment of gum recession. No longer was there an absolute requirement for harvesting the patient's own tissue. In 1997, LifeCell™ introduced acellular dermal matrix (i.e., Alloderm®, etc.) for dental applications. Researchers were able to acquire larger amounts of donor skin tissue in the same way that other organs, such as bone, is acquired. Skin is harvested from people who have designated themselves as donors upon becoming deceased. Once a certified tissue bank has verified through testing that the donor tissue free of diseases (e.g., viruses, etc.), the outer epithelium is removed and the underlying dermis and basement membrane are prepared in such a way that cells are removed but the blood vessels, collagen, elastin, etc., remain. This allows the graft to act as a scaffold for the normal tissue remolding after surgical placement.

And so now, instead of taking tissue from the patient's palate, a periodontist can open up a package of sterilized acellular dermal matrix tissue. The donor tissue graft is prepared then stitched into place and then the patient's gums are stitched up over the top of the graft. This innovation allows periodontists to treat large areas of recession in a single visit with much less discomfort for the patient.

Recently, a newer, less invasive treatment approach for treating gum recession was developed, and this new procedure is now one of our preferred treatment methods. It is called the Chao Pinhole® Surgical Technique (PST™), named for the developer of this proprietary gum recession treatment – Dr. John Chao, DDS, JD.

The PST™ is great because it is a scalpel-free, suture-free procedure, which makes it very appealing for patients. The creative innovation is that, instead of having to loosen the gum tissue right in between the teeth, the periodontist creates tiny pinholes, four to six per jaw, in the mucous membrane. Then, while utilizing specially designed dental instruments, the periodontist gently tunnels and loosens the gum tissue around the tooth and then slides it up along the neck of the tooth. The last step is to place small non-crossed linked collagen under the papillae and along the neck of the teeth.

While this sounds complex, the important thing to know is that the procedure allows your periodontist to treat recession without doing any cutting or stitching, and so there is only minimal, short-term discomfort or swelling for the patient.

My staff and I were trained at the Chao Pinhole Academy near Pasadena, California in 2016, and we really like how our patients have responded to the treatment. Our patients that have opted for the PST™ experience much less discomfort while at the same time we are able to do an even higher quality job of treating the recession. Empirically, I would estimate that patients heal almost twice as fast, as compared to using the traditional gum grafting technique because the papillae remain intact.

New Periodontal Treatments

There are a variety of periodontal treatments available for you, some surgical and some non-surgical, as well as new ways of treating gum disease. Most of the new treatments that have been developed in the past five to ten years are more effective and less invasive, which means that patients heal faster and do not have to deal with as much discomfort, like the PST™ I mentioned earlier.

If you have some mild to moderate level of gum disease that can be easily taken care of with non-surgical treatment, then that is great because you are probably going to heal pretty quickly and be ready sooner for any cosmetic dental procedure. However, it is still going to be probably at least two or three months before all your tissues are completely healed to the point where you are ready to move forward in getting some cosmetic work done. If you have severe periodontal disease, then that healing period is likely going to take a bit longer, even if the periodontist employs one of the newer, less invasive treatments.

One of the newest and most exciting technologies we have been utilizing in our office for more than five years for treating moderate to severe periodontal disease with a unique dental laser. The device is called a PerioLase®. You can probably tell by the name that it is a type of laser that has been specifically developed to treat moderate to severe periodontal disease.

The PerioLase® was created by Millennium Dental Technologies of Cerritos, California, and, honestly, it is revolutionizing how gum disease is treated worldwide. The PerioLase® is used to perform a specific type of Laser Periodontal Therapy™ called Laser Assisted New Attachment Procedure® or LANAP® for short. With LANAP® it is possible to achieve Laser-Assisted Regeneration™ or LAR™. LANAP® is the only FDA-cleared laser to promote True Regeneration™ of the attachment apparatus (new cementum, new periodontal ligament, and new alveolar bone) on a previously diseased root surface when used specifically in the LANAP® Protocol. My staff and I have been specially certified to utilize the PerioLase® and have found it achieves wonderful results for our patients without the need for a scalpel, bone grafting, or stiches.

Is Gum Disease Reversible?

A common question patient have is the question, "Is gum disease reversible?"

Gingivitis, the less severe kind of gum disease is completely reversible with a combination of professional dental cleaning and educating the patient on proper dental care, including daily brushing of the gums, flossing, and using oral rinses.

The more severe kind of gum disease, periodontitis, is not generally reversible without surgical intervention but it can be effectively treated – depending on the severity.

With the most severe cases, there may be nothing your dentist can do to save the tooth, and in those instances, the proper treatment involves talking about tooth removal and tooth replacement such as a dental implant.

Life-Changing Treatment

Let me tell you about one patient I treated, whose case illustrates what a transformational difference getting treated for gum disease can make in a person's life. This was actually a cosmetic case. Maria was in her late twenties when she was referred to me. She had significant gum recession after undergoing orthodontic treatment. Her chief complaint is that, because of her "long tooth" condition, she no longer smiled. She said she was always self-conscious about the way she spoke and laughed because she could see how long her teeth were.

As you can gather, in Maria's situation, the condition of her teeth in relation to her gums was having a severely negative effect on how she lived her daily life and interacted with people. It affected her personal relationships; it affected how she acted at work, and indeed her entire life. Because Maria was so self-conscious and embarrassed about her smile, she was reluctant to socialize with people at all. This was all attributable to gum recession.

We performed extensive gum grafting for her, and the difference was nothing short of miraculous. When she came back to my office for a checkup one month later, she was actually in tears because she was so happy about having regained her self-confidence. It was really remarkable – her whole life changed dramatically for the better in less than a month.

Maria is not alone. I have treated many patients with the same or similar oral conditions. People may not realize what a difference a beautiful smile can make, but I would argue that by getting the proper treatment, you can make your smile, and in effect, your whole face, look 10 or 20 years younger. Periodontal plastic surgery can boost your self-confidence and self-esteem, and that shows through. These procedures have the potential to change everything about a person – how they carry themselves, their facial expressions, and self-confidence.

It can be both shocking and devastating for someone to hear that they have severe periodontal disease. Sometimes certain teeth can be saved, but in some cases, it is recommended to have teeth removed and consider tooth replacement options such as dental implants. Patients need to talk to their dental professional about their options.

As sobering as it may be to hear you need some or all of your teeth removed, we explain the systemic benefits to the patient's overall health. In addition, we discuss tooth replacement options, such as dental implants. We say, "Our goal is to restore balance in your mouth. In time, you will be chewing food like you used to and have a beautiful smile." Restoring balance to chewing while delivering optimal dental esthetics is the ultimate goal for everyone.

I always take the time to explain to patients that it is really important to get treatment because severe periodontal disease can put their whole systemic health at risk. The associations between periodontal disease and systemic diseases – known as the oral-systemic link – are well documented. Your overall systemic health and your oral health often times run hand-in-hand.

One of the most common connections is with diabetes including those pre-diabetic (i.e., glucose intolerance, etc.). People with uncontrolled or poorly controlled diabetes tend to have much more frequent gum disease issues and severity. Of equal importance is that untreated periodontal disease can exacerbate their diabetes condition. Both must be treated to improve the quality and longevity of life for these patients.

Pregnant women with periodontal disease have a higher chance of having a preterm low birth weight baby. Studies show that women that get their periodontal disease under control earlier during their pregnancy have a better chance of their baby being born full term. Also, men with periodontal disease have much higher rates of erectile dysfunction (ED). Studies show that once these men have their periodontal disease effectively treated, most will experience fewer ED issues.

People with active periodontal disease are much more likely to have problems throughout their bodies. Inflammatory mediators and bacteria are constantly entering their bloodstream while targeting the heart and brain. Those with untreated periodontal disease have an increased risk for both heart attack and stroke, as they are all comorbid risk factors in the overall health of a patient. Educating people on the oral-systemic link is a must for each dentist and periodontist. Only well-informed people can be expected to make educated, sometimes life-altering decisions that may affect more than his or her teeth but may also prolong the quality and quantity of life.

Today, most of our patients are very thankful when we can use less invasive procedures, such as the PerioLase® or the Chao Pinhole® Surgical Technique before things become too severe. My patients are thankful and happy not only that we saved their teeth but also because we were able to take a more conservative approach than were possible just a few years ago.

Again, I want to stress that the most important thing is to see your dentist regularly, so that he or she has the opportunity to recognize, at an early stage, any developing problem with gum disease. If you only have gingivitis, then your dentist and dental hygienist can completely treat the areas and give you the knowledge and skills needed to take the best possible care of your teeth to prevent any future problems.

If you have taken the time to read this book, my message to you is simple. I want you to have the best-looking, most attractive smile possible, for your entire life. And there is no reason you cannot have that. In my ideal world, everyone gets proper education on taking care of their teeth and gums, in addition to visiting their dentist twice a year. If your dentist diagnoses you with any form of periodontal disease, it is recommended to see a periodontist as soon as possible. Together, the dentist and periodontist can come up with a plan to restore your dental health and, in many cases, improve your quality of life.

About Bryan P. Kalish, DDS, MS

Implant & Laser Periodontal Surgery Center
www.ElPasoGumSurgery.com

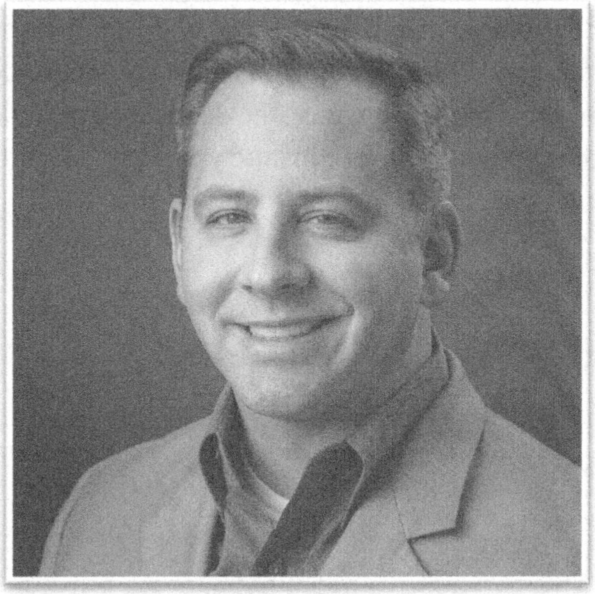

Dr. Bryan P. Kalish has been providing exceptional patient care for nearly a decade and, since his recent retirement from the military, has become part of the El Paso dental community.

As a former periodontal and implant surgery instructor in the United States Army, Dr. Kalish attained the rank of full-bird colonel and received numerous awards and commendations, including the US Army Dental Corps Chief's Exceptional Service and Leadership Award, the US Army Surgeon General's System for Health Gold Award on behalf of the Directorate of Heath Care Operations of the US

Army Dental Command, the Association of Military Surgeons of the United States (AMSUS) Facility Based Healthcare (Hospitals & Clinics) Award on behalf of the US Army Dental Command, and the US Army Surgeon General's "A" Proficiency Designator, which is recognized as the highest level of professional achievement in the US Army Medical Department.

Dr. Kalish specializes in dental implants, bone grafting, and the use of laser and cosmetic periodontal practices. He also specializes in cosmetic lip and cheek injectable fillers, therapeutic Botox to treat TMD and myofascial pain, and the creation of oral sleep appliances.

Dr. Kalish amasses over 100 hours per year of ongoing training. He also travels frequently to demonstrate the most cutting-edge surgical techniques at seminars all over the world, working with other dentists to train them in the latest technology available to help patients receive the highest quality dental care. He has received certificates in Kybella Chin Treatments, Pinhole Surgical Technique, Lip Augmentation and Platelet Rich Plasma Injections, Advanced Botox and Dermal Fillers, and Laser-Assisted New Attachment Procedure® (LANAP) Evolution 5 Proficiency.

Dr. Kalish graduated from college and dental school through the Six-Year Combined BA/DDS program at the University of Missouri – Kansas City (UMKC). He practiced general dentistry in the Army for four years before specializing in dental implants and periodontal surgery. He has worked with patients in Thailand, Korea, Mongolia, Germany, Italy, and Iraq. Today, his passion is to work with patients in the southwestern United States, many of whom travel great distances to receive care from him. A few of his professional accolades include Fellow, Institute for Advanced Laser Dentistry; Fellow, International College of Dentists; Member of the Order of Military Medical Merit; Master in the College of Sedation in Dentistry; Past-President of the European Association of Military Periodontists; Board-Certified Diplomate of the American Board of Periodontology; and membership in the American Board of Periodontology, American Academy of Periodontology, American Academy of Dental Sleep Medicine, American Dental Association, Texas Dental Association, El Paso District Dental Society, Institute for Advanced Laser Dentistry, and International Academy of Facial Aesthetics. He is licensed to practice dentistry is Texas and New Mexico.

Dental Veneers: The Power of Transformation

Your smile is one of the first features people notice upon entering a room. Dental veneers have the amazing ability to enhance your smile aesthetically, as well as strengthen teeth that are compromised.

A dental veneer is a wafer-thin piece of porcelain or ceramic that is used to cover the front of the tooth. It is a beautiful, strong, smooth surface that transforms the outer layer of the tooth. If a tooth is chipped, fractured, or heavily worn down from grinding patterns, veneers can actually strengthen what is lacking or unhealthy.

In addition, veneers can change the look of your teeth dramatically when it comes to shape, texture, or color. They can be applied to one tooth or multiple teeth. This can have life-changing results for people who are unsatisfied or self-conscious about their smile.

One patient in particular comes to mind when I think about the life-changing effects of veneers. A very shy, 27-year-old male stepped into my office. He was mumbling and extremely difficult to understand, though it was not due to an accent or lack of proficiency in the English language. He was simply someone who was too self-conscious to project his own voice.

As the consultation progressed, he revealed to me that the appearance of his teeth was preventing him from getting hired at job interviews. He had an impressive background and education, but cosmetically, he had developed very short teeth over time due to grinding. His grind and wear patterns were so extreme that they resembled the teeth of a 40 to 50-years-old patient. They just didn't match his vibrant, youthful look.

I went ahead and placed 20 veneers, 10 upper and 10 lower teeth. When this young man arrived for his follow-up appointment, he was beaming. He had since been offered his dream job and begun seriously dating a woman he'd met at the interview. The man in front of me was happy, confident, and successful... a true transformation.

He became a regular patient, as we stress the importance of not only making a one-time investment for your teeth but reinvesting to make sure you are achieving optimal oral health. This can be done through cleanings, at least twice annually.

One year later, during his checkup and cleaning, this young man returned and was excited to report he was engaged to be married! I look back on this case and feel an overwhelming sense of pride, knowing we helped him succeed in his career goals and find the love of his life through the power of dental veneers.

Are Dental Veneers for Me?

A typical patient walks through my door for the first time with an aesthetic concern. They aren't going to be so technical as to say, "I don't like my outer enamel." They often describe to me what they see in the mirror, focusing on exactly what is causing them unhappiness or anxiety.

For example, a patient may say, "I don't like the color of my teeth." It is my job to explain to them WHY they see this particular shade and what we can do to improve it. Many times, they have already tried whitening the teeth on their own, and the results simply weren't enough. In this case, they are in search of a more permanent solution.

Other patients arrive with complaints about the texture of their teeth. They may have certain teeth that don't "shine" as much as the others or appear dull and gray. We also see many patients with significant damage to the teeth, whether it be chips from trauma or a sports injury, or heavy grinding and chewing patterns.

Last but not least, there are patients who arrive with a photograph of a Hollywood star and say, "I want my smile to look exactly like this." They don't have a chief complaint about their own smile, but their idol has a better smile and they want the same.

In any of these cases, dental veneers can achieve the desired outcome, creating a happy, healthy, confident patient.

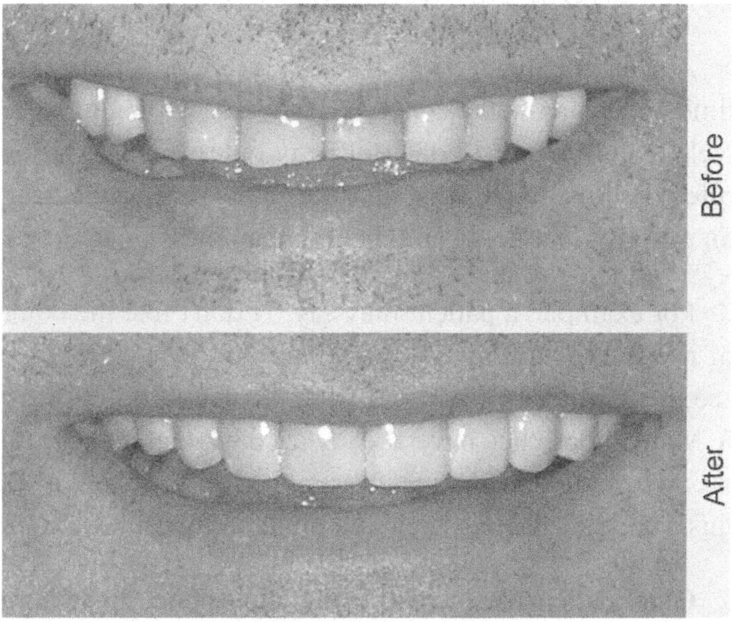

Placing 10 veneers

The Consultation

The first step to any quality procedure is a good, face to face conversation. My goal is to first learn about the patient's chief complaints, as well as financial status. Veneers are an investment, and it is important to discuss this upfront and set realistic expectations. Once the patient has been informed about how veneers will not only correct their chief complaints but also add beauty and life to their smile, they are typically ready to proceed.

At this point, we move to a specialized smile creation technique. I learned this technique from my father, Dr. Gary Davidowitz. He has been practicing for over 45 years in cosmetic dentistry and educating dentists all over the world in the International Aesthetics Department at NYU College of Dentistry. The purpose of this technique is to give the patient an accurate representation of what their "new" smile will look like after the procedure is complete.

We begin by taking detailed photos of the patient with different facial expressions such as a relaxed, close-up smile, and an exaggerated smile. I'm a genuine believer that everyone is truly a nice person, but personalities vary from gruff to gentle. I wouldn't give a very soft and delicate smile to someone with a more aggressive personality. It simply would not match. So that is a very important part of the design factor.

By using the photos and my observations of the patient while speaking with them, I learn about their personality, how they speak, expressions they make, how high their smile arches during a big smile versus a social smile, and so on. I am then able to prescribe and hand draw where I feel the teeth should lie in relation to the face.

All of these observations are taken into consideration and given to the ceramist, who is responsible for creating the veneers. All of this can then be simulated on a computer. The patient can view images of him or herself smiling in different ways, with a whiter smile, wider smile, more length to the teeth, and so on. We can modify the images until the patient is completely satisfied with the vision for the end result.

A digital impression molding is then taken of the teeth, which allows it to be converted to a file for the computer. Using CAD technology, we are able to 3D print these models to the exact proportions we are seeing on the simulation. This is quite remarkable as the patient knows exactly what to expect after the procedure is complete and gets to approve their new smile beforehand.

The Procedure

The procedure begins on the second visit by using a guided template technique. The 3D model consists of just the arches to start, and then we place the wax and veneers on the arches based on the photo simulation. These guided templates are used to carefully and methodically prepare the patient's teeth to accommodate the veneers.

Often, patients develop fear and concern when we talk about "preparing the teeth." The beauty of modern veneers is that not much space is needed as they can be as thin as a contact lens in some areas with a strength that exceeds a natural tooth. As a result, we don't have to drill away at a patient's healthy tooth structure in order to place them. We are simply reshaping the enamel to deliver the results shown on the simulation. A final molding is taken at this point, and the patient is now ready for the placement of temporary veneers.

These temporary veneers are matched to the size and shape of what was seen on the smile simulation and made based upon the guided templates, as discussed above. Then we send the patient off into the world to "test drive" their new smile. How are they living with their new smile? Is there anything about the new smile that feels like it needs modification?

We typically see the patient back again after a few days. If any changes are necessary, I take a new digital impression which can be sent over to the ceramist to show them the exact modifications. The CAD technology is then re-developed to the new shape of the tooth, and 3D printed once more.

On the third visit, the temporary veneers are removed, and the permanent ones are placed. This is referred to as a bonding procedure, the final step of the smile transformation.

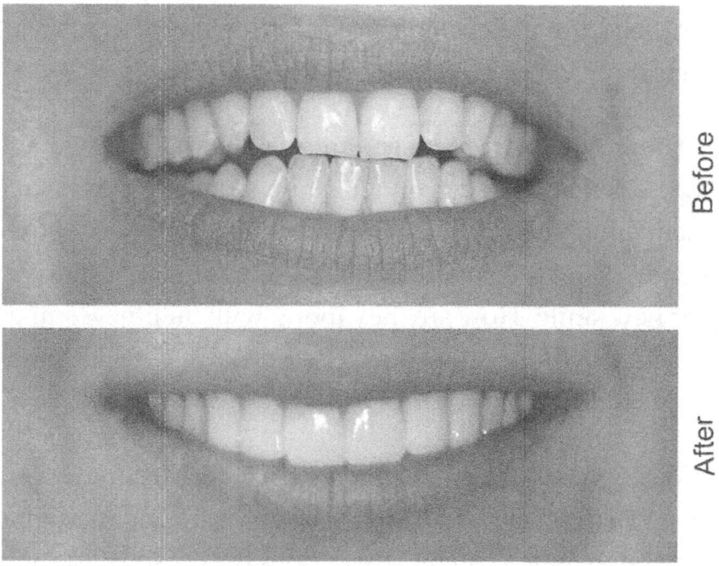

Placing 20 veneers

Types of Veneers

The veneers most commonly used by dentists, as discussed in this chapter, are made of porcelain or ceramic. These are made indirectly, meaning they are processed in a dental laboratory and not made directly in the patient's mouth while in the office.

Another type of veneer is called a resin veneer. These are created using a putty-like resin and freehandedly shaped over the prepared tooth. Once it is shaped accordingly, it is cured by placing a light on it that will immediately harden the material. It is then polished, and the patient is soon sent on their way. This material is not as strong as ceramic, but rather more porous, stains faster, and has a tendency to chip. Ceramic does a better job at mimicking actual enamel.

Another type of veneer is called a prepless veneer. Prepless veneers became popular after a dental laboratory created a porcelain veneer that they claimed could be made as thin as 0.3 millimeters while just as strong as the competition. Today's newer ceramics, however, are strong enough that they could be made to that same minimal thickness.

A prepless veneer is placed over the current tooth structure to improve color, or in some cases, shape. It is more difficult to change shape with this type of veneer since we are not altering the original tooth in any way. The only likely candidates for prepless veneers would be those who have very "flat profile" teeth, preventing the veneers from looking bulky or oversized. Therefore, prepless veneers are the least commonly used.

It is important to remember that "one size does not fit all" when it comes to veneers. Even amongst ceramic veneers, there are many different types. The reason for using one over another is really up to the dentist.

I will consider factors like how much tooth structure remains, the current color and shade of the tooth, and what kind of force relationship exists in the patient's mouth. For example, the type of veneer that we use on somebody who is a severe clencher is going to be different than somebody who has very little muscle mass of the jaw and no sign of wear and tear on the teeth.

A skilled cosmetic dentist can advise you on the best veneers for your particular needs.

The Benefits of Veneers Over Teeth Whitening

As an experienced cosmetic dentist, I am rarely surprised when patients express some form of disappointment with the results of bleaching. They will agree that the teeth look brighter. They leave the office generally happy, but then disappointment sets in. And it's not that the bleach didn't work. I personally use a *Zoom* teeth whitening by Philips, which yields great results and can produce a bright and natural whiteness, at least during the short term.

But more often than not, people realize they want much more than that. They sometimes focus so much on the color that they get distracted from the bigger picture: the complete smile. Elements such as shape, contour, and harmony of the teeth in relationship to the lips and face are just as significant as color. So these elements produce an aesthetic effect greater than the sum of its parts.

Traditional whitening is only good for a certain amount of time before the teeth become stained again from regular use. Patients will need to repeat the treatment, especially if they are smokers, coffee drinkers, or simply have teeth that are predisposed to staining. For a one-time investment, porcelain veneers will remain virtually stain-free and bright for the entire life of the veneer – an average of 15-20 years.

Another disadvantage of traditional whitening is a condition known as "bleaching anorexia." This refers to the constant exposure of bleach to a tooth over a period of time, causing harm to the enamel and resulting in a hypersensitive tooth.

Also, consider that traditional whitening methods will not be able to whiten inorganic material such as crowns or fillings. This will result in a terrible mismatch of brightness and color from tooth to tooth. Veneers allow for uniform color and shading throughout the entire mouth.

Veneers and Orthodontics

In the case of a patient with overcrowded teeth, there is a great benefit to straightening the teeth before placing veneers. There are two major benefits to getting orthodontic work done before getting veneers. First of all, straight teeth automatically translate to healthier gums. When teeth are overlapping, it constricts the health of the gums and makes those areas more difficult to clean. Masking these areas with veneers is not going to accomplish a positive long-term result.

Secondly, teeth that are already straight require minimal preparation on my end to be ready for the veneers. As discussed previously, preserving as much of the tooth structure as possible is always my main goal.

In situations where there is only minor crowding, a little bit of overlap, or a little relapse from past orthodontics, I would recommend going straight to veneers. In these cases, the teeth have already settled into a position where they are happy. We would still keep our minimal conservative dentistry approach.

Veneers can provide an "instant orthodontics" for patients with slight crowding. Once the veneers are properly prepared and placed, it will look like you have completed orthodontics in just a couple of weeks!

Veneers in Conjunction with Other Dental Procedures

Some patients may benefit from specific cosmetic or restorative procedures prior to placing veneers. I often recommend whitening the teeth before the veneer procedure. Veneers are like glass and have a very translucent quality. The brighter we can make the teeth beforehand, the better.

In cases of restorative work, some patients already have crowns on some of their teeth. We would typically remove those crowns and match new ones to the particular veneer ceramic being used. We would treat a patient with a missing tooth in the same manner, matching the implant with the veneering. In this way, veneers and existing crowns or implants flow seamlessly together, creating a uniform, beautiful smile.

There are instances where gum reshaping can greatly enhance the beauty of veneers. For instance, a "gummy smile" can be reduced with the use of dental lasers prior to veneer placement.

Common Myths About Veneers

Myth #1: Veneers are only needed for the front teeth.

The number of veneers is determined by many factors, number one being the chief complaints of the patient. Will placing veneers on just the four front teeth satisfy the patient's chief complaints? And if so, how is the rest of the smile going to look? If a patient asks me to only place veneers on the front teeth, it is my responsibility to determine whether or not those four veneers will fit well with the rest of their smile.

Myth #2: Veneers look "fake."

Some patients have preconceived notions about how veneers will appear after the procedure is complete. They may have seen people with veneers that appear "fake," and do not want that to be the case for themselves. Veneers should not look fake. It comes down to the design, what materials are being used, who the dentist decides to collaborate with on a laboratory basis, and, of course, the patient's desires. Veneers can be made to look as natural as can be, even having imperfections built in. The look of the veneer, whether "perfect" or "natural," is completely up to the patient.

Myth #3: Getting veneers is painful.

Many people associate getting veneers with painful drilling and tooth sensitivity. As mentioned throughout this chapter, I want to preserve as much of the natural tooth structure as possible. This translates to MINIMAL removal of tooth structure, even less than with a filling or crown. As with any typical dental procedure, a local anesthetic is used so that the patient does not feel any part of the tooth preparation process. Placing veneers is a painless procedure that gives amazing, long-lasting results.

Myth #4: Veneers are only used for aesthetic purposes.

There are situations where veneers are not just an aesthetic proponent but also a way of fortifying weakened teeth. Some people are born with unhealthy enamel. Their teeth are more porous, which makes them more prone to staining and cavities. Some of those same people have needed fillings on their front teeth and yet, those fillings are not holding up. They become discolored and chipped. Putting porcelain over these surfaces will not only beautify them but protect them from further degradation.

Other instances are those who grind their teeth or who have chipped their teeth due to injury. They may have tried other alternatives like bonding, using a resin to repair the tooth, though it quickly starts to feel like a constant battle, requiring consistent repair. A veneer will restoratively fix that problem. It will build back the tooth in a stronger fashion than the other options and as a bonus, you get cosmetic benefits.

Myth #5: Veneers are likely to break or chip.

Although veneers are very thin, they are amazingly strong and will not break or chip easily. And while it's important to exercise common sense, regular eating such as biting into a bagel, a sandwich, or a carrot can be done without risk. Remember that with veneers, the ceramic that we are using is stronger than enamel. The bond that ceramic has to our teeth is tremendously strong.

A skilled cosmetic dentist is keenly aware of the biting forces of each individual patient. The only problems that should ever arise when it comes to chipping or breaking are the result of veneers that were not properly designed in the first place. A patient who is a heavy grinder will require a much different design than one who is not. This is why it is so important to find a knowledgeable, experienced professional that you feel comfortable with.

Common Mistakes

Mistake #1: Wrong Color

People always want their teeth to look natural, but really white, which is actually a contradiction. Teeth are either yellow-white or gray-white by nature. They are never white-white by nature. The trick is making the teeth appear white without appearing dense, opaque, and fake. I would never want a patient to walk out after a smile makeover and look like they have dentures. Denture teeth are opaque and dense. Veneers are life-like.

The nice thing about the newer materials is that we are able to create a balance between natural and white. We can create a very nice, white smile but still have the translucency. We want the veneers to absorb some of the light and still look natural.

Even if a patient requests "paper-white" teeth, we'll have a long conversation about why that may not be the best idea. Skin tone and whites of eyes play a large role in the color of the veneers I choose for the patient. Fair-skinned people can go with whiter shades. Similarly, people with more white than gray in the whites of their eyes look better with whiter shades of veneers.

Mistake #2: Wrong Number

Placing too few veneers can often lead to a disappointed patient. As discussed previously, the number of veneers placed should not only fix the chief complaints of the patient, but create a uniform, beautiful smile in harmony with the rest of the teeth. We would only choose to place a small number of veneers if those matched perfectly with the existing teeth.

There are also patients who request just a top arch or a bottom arch. Though we see more of the top arch when we smile, we see more of the bottom arch when we speak. Therefore, consistency between the two is also essential. If a patient is not ready to make the jump to top and bottom all at once, we typically start with the top since the "curtains go up when we smile." Since the lower lip hides much of the anatomy of the lower teeth, lower veneers are not a necessity. In any case, top and bottom placement will always result in a complementary, uniform smile.

How Much Do Veneers Cost?

The cost of veneers varies based upon the dentist, laboratory, and location. But a typical price range is $2,000 to $3,000 per veneer. This price range is affected by a couple of factors. The first one is geographic location. It is dependent on where in the country you get the work done and how much it costs to maintain and run an office and lab in that area.

Secondly, quality comes into play. I would be very wary of the lower end cost on a veneer because I know the importance of choosing the right partner in a dental laboratory. The materials used and the artistry and commitment need to be top-notch. This results in constant success in veneer treatment.

The importance of seeing somebody who has experience is half the battle. That same person has to be working in conjunction with a quality dental laboratory that is working behind the scenes. The ceramicist can make or break a perfectly planned and executed case and the final treatment outcome. So the proper collaboration is crucial. "You get what you pay for" rings true when it comes to dental veneers.

One story stands out in my mind when it comes to the importance of choosing an experienced cosmetic dentist. A young woman came into my office for the consultation. I asked her what her chief complaints were, and she started tearing up. I said, "Let me just take a look. Give me a smile." I could hardly see anything because her lips were so tightly wound around the teeth that it was impossible to evaluate what was going on.

The cause of her embarrassment, unfortunately, was having veneers placed incorrectly and with terrible discoloration. The gums were very red and inflamed, and her adjacent teeth were actually very white, almost bleached white. I asked her who had performed this work. It was done by her long-time dentist, who had performed the work three times, with the results worse and worse each time.

Upon further evaluation, I determined there were several issues: the thickness of the veneer, the condition of the gums, the discoloration of the veneers, and the number of veneers placed. There were only three veneers placed in front, which is an odd number. Without symmetry, that number would never look right. So we decided to add one. The rest of her teeth were absolutely beautiful.

We moved on with the treatment plan and she was able to see her new smile on the simulation screen. We waxed up four new veneers and removed the old ones. We cleaned up the gums nicely since they were very inflamed; this was due to the improper thickness of the old veneers at the gumline. With the placement of just those four brand new veneers, her smile was once again beautiful. Her smile was always beautiful, of course, but had been compromised by a dentist who lacked the necessary experience.

When she came back for her follow-up appointment, her stunning smile was on showcase. She was feeling wonderful, no adjustments were needed, and she had regained her confidence.

After this experience, as well as countless others, I feel fortunate to have the ability to create unique, carefully considered plans and execute them in a way that changes people's lives through the power of dental veneers.

About Steven Davidowitz, DDS

Luxury Dental NYC
www.LuxuryDentistryNYC.com

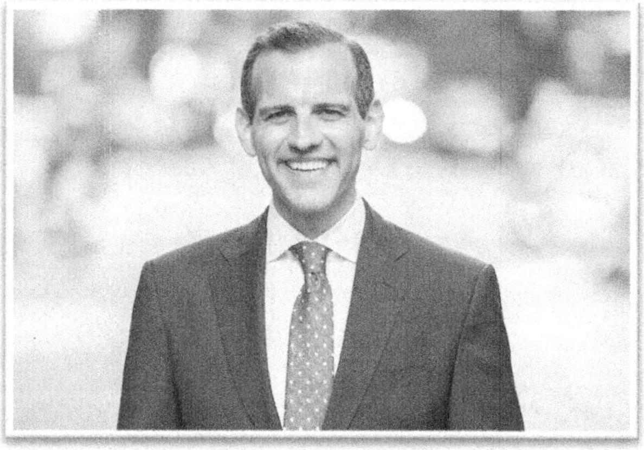

Dr. Steven Davidowitz, also known as "Dr. D" by his patients, is the owner and practicing dentist at Luxury Dentistry NYC located in the UES of Manhattan.

Dr. Steven received his DDS degree from the New York University College of Dentistry and completed a general dentistry residency at the Brooklyn Hospital Medical Center. He did his fellowship training in Implant Surgery and Restorative Implant Dentistry at New York University and is a Fellow in International Congress of Oral Implantologists.

Dr. Steven practices general and cosmetic dentistry with a true love for smile makeovers through clear aligner and porcelain veneer treatment. Dr. Steven is also a Co-Founder and serves as the Director of Dental Services at MOD Mouth.

Dr. Steven is an active member in the American Academy of Clear Aligners (AACO) in which he has published multiple articles on clear aligner therapy and modalities. As well as, being a member of the American Dental Association (ADA), the Academy of General Dentistry (AGD), and the American Academy of Facial Esthetics (AAFE).

He was recently named a member of the RealSelf Medical Review Advisory Board for cosmetic dentistry content on their website and platform at realself.com.

Dr. Steven is also an official sponsor and supporter of "Women Of Wall Street" a Global Private Society of influential women in different industries and job titles ranging from Writers, to VPs of Finance Firms, Investors, Award Winning Producers, Media Personalities, Scientists and more.

Dr. Steven lives in Woodmere, NY. He is married to Shana Davidowitz a practicing Nurse Practitioner of Women's Health at Northwell Health - LIJ. They have two children together, Eli and Lily.

DR. MARIANA CONANT

Biting Right is Biting Tight

Many dental patients are primarily focused on esthetics when it comes to their teeth and smile. Usually what they see is what matters most. When they see that their front teeth are chipped, they often want these repaired first. However, a good question a patient could be asking their dentist is, "Why are my teeth chipping?" Also, they need to ask their dentist, "How can I avoid this from happening again in the future?"

The answer requires a detailed exam making sure teeth, gums and tissues are healthy, the bite is stable and the temporomandibular joint (TMJ—which is a hinge-like connection on either side of the head that allows the lower jaw to move) is also stable. If only the front teeth are addressed—the ones that are visible to the patient and others—and the TMJ and bite aren't considered, any treatment the patient receives may not be long-lasting.

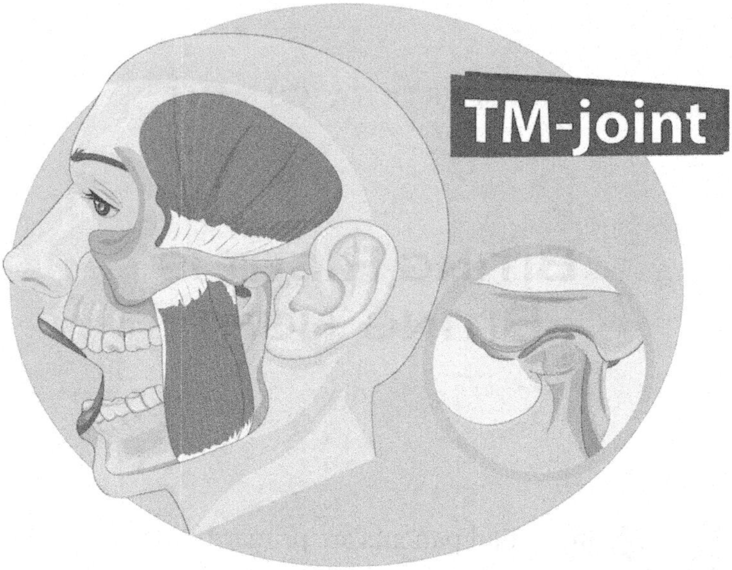

What Do We Mean by a Stable Bite?

A stable bite can be defined as the teeth closing together properly. The upper teeth should fit slightly over the lower teeth and the points of the back teeth ideally fit inside the grooves of their opposing teeth in such a way that the jaw muscles are relaxed and comfortable, forces are well distributed, the TMJ is not under pressure, and chewing is easy. A good bite promotes less wear on the teeth, so they break less, last longer and look younger as we age.

When a bite is out of alignment, we can look at it from two viewpoints. Poor alignment can affect facial esthetics as well as overall functionality. From an esthetic point of view, when the bite is off, we may notice facial asymmetry and the smile may look crooked because the teeth do not close together properly.

The second consideration is functionality, and this can range from mild to severe. For example, dysfunction in the TMJ may cause what is called trismus, which means the jaw gets locked. As you can imagine, this is an alarming situation.

I had a patient, age 32, who arrived at the office in tremendous pain, he could not talk. His jaw had dislocated and was now locked. I was able to manipulate his jaw back into place. He was tremendously relieved. He also wanted to never have to go through that experience again, and that's what I will be talking about in this chapter—how to prevent TMJ problems as well as how to improve the esthetics of your smile in a healthy way.

Sometimes, bite problems are not so apparent and it is easier for a dentist to detect them like tooth wear, cracks and fractures. More visible issues like a crossbite—when a tooth is positioned more towards the cheek or the tongue then it should, narrow arches, open bite, overbite (deep bite), or an underbite—which means the lower jaw and teeth extend beyond the upper teeth, require orthodontic evaluation and treatment.

The esthetic aspect is one thing, and that can affect a person's life, but problems that aren't visible can do that as well. TMJ disorder, also known as temporomandibular disorder (TMD), can be associated with the way the upper and the lower teeth fit together, but also with headaches, including migraines for example, jaw locking, painful clicking and popping of the jaw, ear pain, facial muscle pain, neck pain, shoulder pain and muscle spasms. Even lower back pain has been reported. On the other hand, jaw clicking or popping alone, without pain or compromised jaw movement, does not indicate a TMJ disorder and does not require treatment.

If the teeth aren't aligned correctly, the tooth to tooth contact isn't harmonious and the biting forces are not distributed equally between the upper and lower teeth when the patient bites down. This can cause pain in specific teeth or radiated pain to other parts of the mouth, head and body.

When a person bites down, this represents a force of 160 pounds per square inch, on average. When the bite is good, that force is distributed evenly on all teeth. However, biting down with this kind of force can cause microfractures in the teeth as well as wear even if the bite is well-aligned. When the bite is out of alignment, this force can cause restorations, fillings, crowns, and even teeth to fracture more easily. So, if a filling or crown needs to be replaced, the patient's bite needs to be evaluated.

Let's say a patient comes in with a cracked tooth. If the bite isn't well balanced, putting a crown on that tooth might not solve the problem. In other words, if an unstable bite contributed for the tooth to crack, that can result in additional fractures. The root cause of that one tooth breaking may be that the bite is off.

WHAT IS TMD?

TMD is a group of conditions that cause dysfunction and pain in the TMJ and on the muscles that control jaw movement. It is a problem that occurs in the intricate area of the jaw located just in front of the ears. The TMJ is located bilaterally where the temporal bone, which is on the lateral side and base of the skull, meets the mandible—the lower jawbone. In between where these two bones meet is a small disc made of fibrocartilage.

Synovial fluid lubricates the joint and protects the disc.

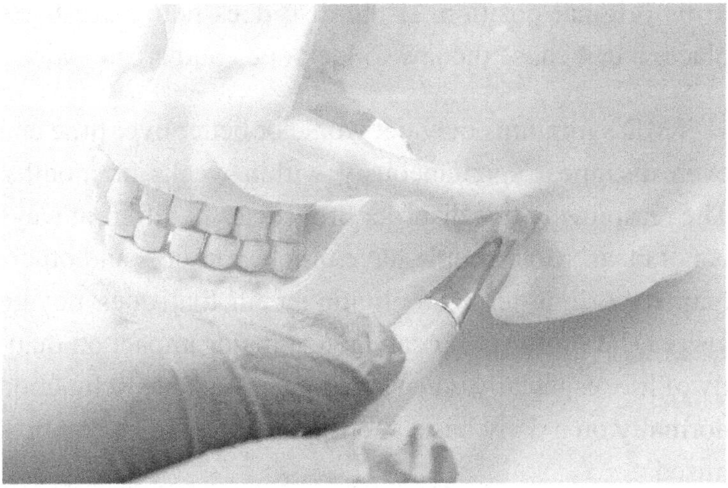

The jawbone is the largest, strongest and lowest bone of the face. There's a small rounded area at the top of the jawbone called the condyle. The condyle slides as the jaw is opened, closed, moved forward, back or sideways. The disc provides a cushion acting as a shock absorber. If that disc becomes displaced or damaged, it may cause TMD. TMD may originate from a problem in the TMJ itself, injury, dislocation, tooth and jaw alignment, grinding, problems in the muscles surrounding the joint or from arthritis.

If the temporal bone, the mandible bone, and the disc in between them aren't in harmony, this can cause the disc to slip out and the jaw apparatus to dislodge. When the disc slips out, usually anteriorly, we call it an anterior disc displacement. This may result in a range of signs and symptoms—from clicking and popping sounds when the jaw is opened to severe discomfort. The disc is a delicate structure and if it gets dislodged, it may or may not return to its original position. If the disc does not return to its place, it can cause the jaw to lock open and create pain.

TMD symptoms may get worse or better over time and even disappear spontaneously within weeks or months. The reason why this disorder progresses in different ways is not clear. Most people have mild symptoms and others may have long-term debilitating pain that does not go away. Therefore, TMD can have a major impact on quality of life, especially when someone is not able to function normally on a daily basis and regular chewing is compromised.

Problems Caused by a Bite That is Out of Alignment

An unstable bite creates problems in the TMJ that cause the jaw to move in inappropriate ways. This results in excessive pressure on the teeth, muscles, TMJ, and even the disc, which in turn can cause the teeth to wear excessively and fracture and the supporting tissues to break down.

There's nothing more dynamic in the body than the mouth. Our mouths are often in motion—from ordinary movements like chewing, yawning and speaking to damaging jaw movements like grinding while asleep. We open and close our mouths several times a day which makes the TMJ the most used joint in the body.

All these things put a great deal of stress on the teeth and, consequently, on the jaw and the TMJ. So, a stable TMJ and a stable bite are essential to prevent damage and pain.

A good analogy for poor alignment of the teeth and jaw is a table with four legs. If one leg is shorter than the other three, the table is going to be unstable, and this will compromise the integrity of the whole table. In the same way, whatever is causing misalignment of the teeth must be resolved, or a TMD may set in.

As mentioned before, it is necessary to look at the whole picture before we start to treat one tooth. Sometimes, the solution is simple. If there's a lot of tooth wear that's causing the teeth to become shorter—which changes the appearance of the face—a little composite can be applied to the canine teeth to make them rise the way they should. This will help protect the back teeth as well as the front teeth from cracking or wearing down even more. If the canines are excessively worn, their heights need to be reestablished. This is often one of the simplest and most efficient methods for protecting the teeth and easing discomfort in the TMJ.

If a patient needs a crown due to a fractured tooth, we need to recognize that when there is a problem with a single tooth, we need to evaluate the TMJ and the relationship between the upper and the lower teeth when they contact to make sure the bite is well aligned. One of the reasons for ongoing tooth problems—like wearing and breakage—is not recognizing all these multiple, negative factors that may be affecting the teeth.

Correcting a Bite That is Out of Alignment

Before balancing an uneven bite, we need to make sure there is no need for orthodontic treatment. Then, the first step would be to do a bite analysis. The dentist will take impressions, create models of the patient's teeth, collect data, and analyze the models to discover the first point of contact. The models give the dentist a blueprint to work from to determine what can be done to improve the bite. From there the bite can be equilibrated with selective tooth grinding in order to improve tooth contact patterns and achieve a stable bite. A sequence is created and then transferred to the patient's teeth by performing what is called an occlusal adjustment (bite adjustment). This is an irreversible procedure and must be done very carefully.

When an occlusal adjustment is performed, we dentists will remove interferences that keep the teeth from closing together properly little by little until the bite is stable. We can create a bite that is more comfortable, and this results in longer-lasting teeth, because they are more protected from damage. It also promotes a healthier TMJ.

Additionally, these adjustments may also require the addition of composite resin filling material to the teeth if the bite isn't too compromised and the teeth aren't severely broken or damaged. If there's extensive damage, the affected teeth may be reconstructed with crowns and veneers, sometimes called a smile makeover or a full mouth reconstruction.

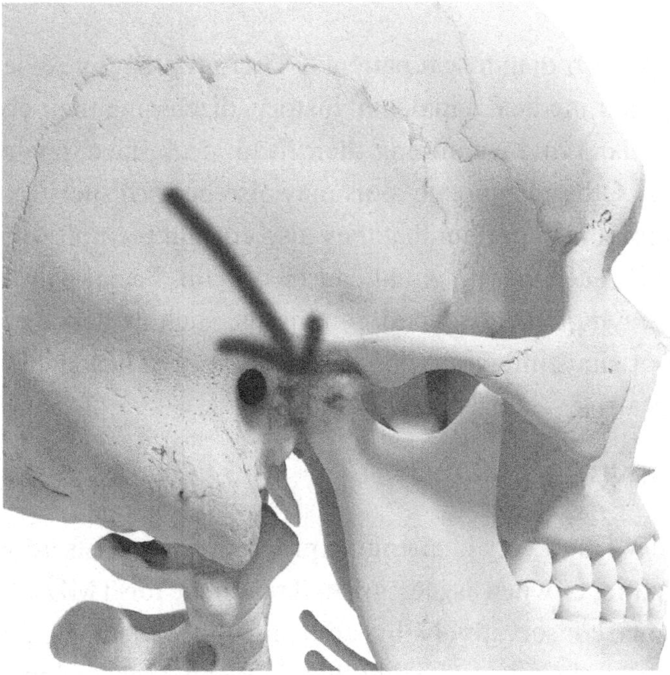

How to Know if You Have a TMJ Problem

Usually, people are only aware of a possible TMJ issue if they hear clicking or popping in the jaw, their jaw dislocates or it develops pain. When the jaw starts hurting, it is more difficult to treat. Some of these cases resolve on their own because the disc has the ability to adapt to a new situation over time. But if a TMD reaches an advanced stage, sometimes the only option is to relieve the pain. It's possible for the jaw to feel better, but the dysfunction may not be corrected.

We can diagnose a patient's TMJ problem by reviewing their medical and dental history, discussing their chief complaint and examining their head, neck, face, jaw and teeth. Other diagnostic tools may also be used such as imaging. It is important that they also consult their physician to rule out other potential causes of pain. Facial pain can be a symptom of several conditions, such as nerve pain, ear or sinus infections and different types of headaches or migraines.

Treating TMD

TMD is a very challenging problem for dentists as well as patients when issues arise. Treatment for TMD often begins conservatively by advising the patient to avoid opening their jaw so wide that they can hear clicking or popping in an effort to prevent the disc from becoming dislodged. The goal is to relax and rest the lower jaw as much as possible. If the patient has acute pain we recommend eating softer foods, taking over the counter medications that reduce inflammation, using warm compresses and practicing relaxation. Most TMJ problems are temporary and these simple steps in treatment would be enough to relieve discomfort.

Some patients with TMD are recommended an occlusal splint therapy by utilizing a custom-made oral appliance made of plastic or acrylic material that fits over the teeth either in the upper or the lower jaw.

An occlusal splint is designed to bring the TMJ to its most comfortable position by changing the bite relationship. A splint is specifically designed for each individual patient, it protects the teeth and jaws from the adverse effects of grinding and clenching (bruxism) and prevents muscle tension and pain. It does not eliminate bruxism but rather distributes the biting forces evenly. It is also recommended prior to extensive restorative work. Once the patient is comfortable in their new position, the dentist can either perform a full mouth reconstruction or orthodontic treatment.

With teeth that have advanced wear and tear, we lose what is called the vertical dimension of occlusion—the superior-inferior relationship of the upper and lower jaws. At this point, it may be required to restore the vertical dimension with crowns and possibly veneers. Sometimes when teeth are missing, implant restorations or bridges are also necessary to reestablish the height lost from the teeth being worn down making sure all restorations meet each other well when the upper and lower teeth touch and also that they do not interfere with each other during regular movements.

Another type of appliance is called the NTI. It is a small custom fit device that fits over the patient's front teeth. It is recommended for cases of frequent migraines or headaches caused by involuntary clenching and grinding. Bruxism will cause the muscles around the jaw to become hyperactive and this leads to headaches and migraines as well as tooth damage, jaw pain and neck pain. The NTI works by preventing the back teeth from contacting and allowing the TMJ and the muscles to relax. It stops the pain and protects the teeth from excessive wear.

A diagnosis from your dentist will determine which type of appliance is indicated, when it needs to be worn and for how long.

The above treatments offer a temporary relief and are not to be considered a cure for TMD. Make sure you visit your dentist regularly and if the symptoms persist, keep them informed. If none of the previous treatments are effective, it may be necessary to have a team of experts involved in diagnosing and treating this condition, such as an ENT specialist, a rheumatologist, a neurologist and a pain management doctor. TMJ surgery is irreversible and should be avoided when possible.

How Much Does It Cost to Treat TMD?

The cost of treating TMD depends on a number of factors including geographic location, the doctor's expertise, and the extent of the work that needs to be done. In my experience, an appliance may cost anywhere between $500 and $3500.

How to Prevent TMD

There are a number of things patients can do to prevent TMJ problems. These are the habits to avoid: chewing on ice, chewing gum, biting your nails or objects, opening your jaw too wide while yawning or singing, resting your chin on your hand, eating hard or crunchy foods that require chewing forcefully. And try sleeping on your back, practicing relaxation and maintaining good posture.

Lastly, people under stress tend to clench their teeth involuntarily. Sometimes, we can tell that we were clenching when we notice generalized tenderness or pain in the jaw bone. There is a mantra I teach my patients to think about daily: "Lips together, teeth apart." That's the key. Be mindful at all times of keeping your jaw relaxed so this becomes a habit.

How Treatment for TMD or Bite Problems Can Change Your Life

Comprehensive dental exam and tailored treatment is paramount. For instance, I have a patient who came in with constant overwhelming migraines. She is a teacher, 55 years of age, and, because of the pain, she couldn't function anymore. She stated she could no longer focus on her job and take care of her family. I did an exam and found she had a great deal of gum recession associated with grinding. This recession had created severe sensitivity, because most of the roots of her teeth were exposed, and there were deep notches on her teeth by the gumline. The roots of our teeth are not meant to be exposed and when that happens, these notches can form which are damaging and our teeth can begin to deteriorate if the issue is not addressed.

We made her an NTI appliance to alleviate the intense pain she was having and restored her notched teeth with composite resin to the root surfaces that had minor gum recession. Where significant areas of gum recession were present, gingival grafts were performed by her periodontist. After the acute pain was under control, we fabricated a custom-made splint for her so she could sleep peacefully. The patient said this treatment changed her life. She has been able to sleep and function normally, and now she feels like a different person.

My goal is to empower patients through education and help improve the quality of life of those affected by these conditions. What I enjoy most is actually seeing all the positive changes in our patients' lives. It is so rewarding to give patients peace of mind with dental restorations that are both functional and beautiful.

About Mariana Conant, DDS

Smile Esthetics Scottsdale
www.SmileEsthetics.com

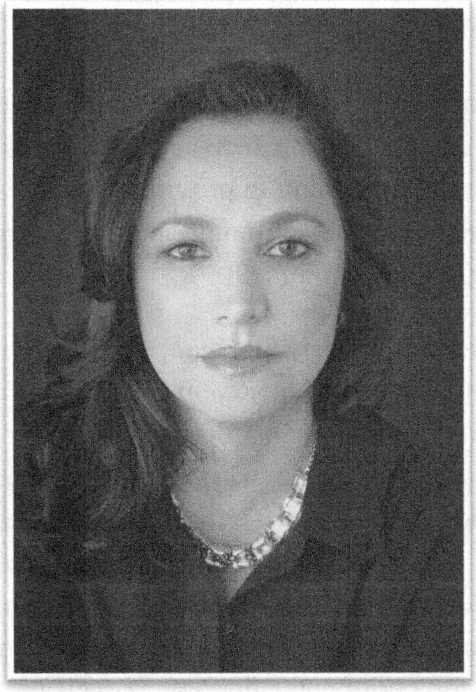

Dr. Mariana Conant received her first DDS degree at Universidade Federal de Goiás, Brazil, in 1997 where she participated in the university's TMJ research with concentration on the diagnosis and treatment of temporomandibular disorders. Dr. Conant is also a 2005 graduate of New York University College of Dentistry, New York City, where she received her second DDS degree and participated in the prestigious Aesthetics Honors Program during her senior year.

She has also completed countless hours of professional study in several areas of dentistry. Dr. Conant focuses her practice on evidence-based esthetic dentistry in order to provide her patients with proper occlusion, ideal function and overall wellness.

Her dental office provides a pleasant and comfortable atmosphere where patients feel welcome. She is diligent in her pursuit to stay current in providing the latest in dental care procedures while utilizing state-of-the-art technology, materials and equipment.

Dr. Conant has received advanced training in comprehensive and implant dentistry in order to assist patients with severely compromised dentition. She provides cosmetic dentistry including whitening, porcelain veneers, esthetic-looking crowns, dentures and bridges. She has had years of experience with short-term orthodontics, such as clear aligner therapy and also clear braces. She offers gum recession treatment, extractions, non-surgical treatment for periodontal disease as well as preventive care and education.

Dr. Conant is a member of the Omicron Kappa Upsilon National Dental Honor Society which represents the highest standards of dentistry. She also received the NYU clinic award for superior performance in providing oral comprehensive care and managing a dental practice. Dr. Conant provides quality dentistry for her patients, caring for adults and children of all ages. She is widely recognized for her thorough and gentle care.

Let's Get Something Straight: Orthodontics

Orthodontics is an important aspect of cosmetic dentistry. An orthodontist is a highly-trained specialist who moves teeth to correct misalignment or (malocclusions) improper bites. Having teeth that are properly aligned and fit appropriately are key to overall oral health to having a great smile and enhancing your facial esthetics.

Traditional orthodontic treatment involves the use of braces. Functionally, braces will correct a bite problem resulting from teeth being crooked or otherwise out of proper alignment, and of course, they can also serve the cosmetic purpose of giving you a more attractive smile.

Today, more and more people are very interested in health, in beauty, and their own personal looks. People very much want to look good, feel good and be healthy, and part of that is having perfectly straight teeth for a beautiful "Hollywood smile."

As orthodontists, we want your arches, which means your upper and lower jaw shape, perfectly aligned and fitting together, for comfort, stability, function, health and of course, cosmetic purposes as well.

The braces themselves are actually “small handles” that we glue to the teeth. In the old days, we used metal braces. We advanced later to using ceramic braces. Braces, whether ceramic or metal look like little squares glued on your teeth.

It is the wires that we tie into the braces that supply the force that gets the teeth moving in the desired direction. There are different types of braces, some of which have less friction and move the teeth faster or easier, and there are others that have programmed slots that receive the wires. It used to be the wires that really did all the work. Within the last ten years due to different bracket design and materials the brackets do some of the work as well. With braces the overall process uses varying forces that are delivered through the bracket, the bracket doors (for self-ligating brackets), the wires and the ligation and other auxiliaries utilized

There are braces that actually self-tie themselves in with doors that hinge closed over the wire, and there are braces that you tie the wire(ligate) in using elastic o-rings. The o-rings come clear, but they also come in a variety of colors, which is something that a lot of kids like.

Braces for Children

We generally don't look to do orthodontic treatments before the age of seven. If you start any earlier than that, then there just usually aren't enough permanent teeth present for you to really create any significant improvement. But we do like to see children around that age so that if there are some developing problems, we can catch and treat them early enough to prevent the need for more extensive treatment such as extractions or jaw surgery.

Even though most children do not need treatments then, they should still be screened because you just don't know who does need treatment unless you are able to check them. That's the reason that we (and the AAO) recommend every child be screened early, by age 7.

For patients who do need treatment, we always try to time the start of treatment as efficiently as possible. That way the treatment doesn't take any longer than necessary. With wires that move faster and faster today, if you put braces on too soon, then it doesn't mean that the patient will get the braces off sooner – instead, it just means that they're going to have the braces on for longer time.

Treatment with Braces

As far as how long treatment does take, that can vary widely from one patient to another, depending on the patient's diagnosis, and treatment plan. A number of factors can play into that, such as how much tooth movement required, how much jaw growth or jaw (orthopedic) correction is necessary, just how each patient responds to treatment along with various habits or airway issues. We've had patients that needed as little as three months of orthodontic treatment, and other patients who needed treatment for up to two and a half years.

The required treatment time can also vary depending on what the patient's expressed desires are about what they would like us to do for them. A simple one tooth cross bite may take a lot less time than treatment designed to achieve an overall comprehensive result that includes not only great function but also ideal cosmetic results. This latter scenario usually includes precise tooth measurements and the collaboration of an excellent cosmetic dentist and periodontist as well. In this manner, the shape, size, position, emergence profile, incisal display, gingival relation, lip fullness and relation are all recognized, diagnosed and intimately addressed!

The necessary frequency of office visits during treatment is also something that varies from patient to patient, depending on the nature of the treatment and how the individual patient responds. If we're doing orthopedic treatment on the jaw, office visits may vary greatly.

When talking about (dentofacial) orthopedic treatment, there are cases where we may need to develop a patient's upper and lower jaws a bit more to create sufficient space so that there's a better chance of avoiding adult teeth extractions later.

It is very important to treat children while they're young and still growing, dentofacial orthopedic work on the jaws is very important in preventing more invasive procedures later.

We can widen jaws with orthopedic movements. We can also maximize the jaw's genetic growth potential by placing the jaws in certain positions that stimulate jaw growth. There are now special appliances that we can have custom fabricated which attach to the teeth and will begin to either expand or advance the jaws in certain positions that stimulate muscle and bone growth, thereby obviating any orthopedic disharmony resulting in a great profile without surgery! A BIG WIN!

By working both on the position and shape of the jaws, along with straightening the patient's teeth, we can dramatically improve someone's appearance, and the overall look of their face. Facial appearance shows improvement, also their profile, and at the same time the alignment of their teeth.

For general orthodontic treatment with braces, we typically only need to see patients about once every eight to ten weeks. We don't usually need to see patients with braces as often as we did in the past, thanks to developing more advanced wires that keep the teeth moving over a longer time without needing adjustments. That's really an important advance because it means patients don't have to come in as often and miss work or school as often as was the case in the past. Additionally, there is MUCH less discomfort with the newer futuristic wires.

We do want to also check patients regularly to see if they're having any particular problems with discomfort. Some patients are apprehensive about pain or discomfort from wearing braces. We try to allay those concerns by using the analogy of having a bruise. It's sort of like having a bruise on your arm. It doesn't hurt all the time, but if you press on it, it definitely feels tender or sore. In the same way, when you put pressure on your teeth by biting, especially right after having your braces tightened up, then you're going to feel some soreness.

But it's not like walking around with a severe toothache all day. It's just the normal inflammatory and healing response that comes from the fact that we are gradually moving the actual roots of the teeth through the jaw bone.

Maintenance of Braces

We recommend patients keep their braces clean through normal, good oral hygiene using a toothbrush, toothpaste, flossing, electric toothbrushes, or a Waterpik or similar device. With children, we tell parents to basically use anything that will help motivate your child to keep their teeth clean. Simple frequent brushing and flossing are just as good as anything as long as they're done properly. We do spend a lot of time teaching and educating patients about how to take care of their teeth.

We also recommend prescription strength fluoride rinse to keep the enamel hard and resistant to cavities. Other than that, just brushing with regular toothpaste with fluoride works great.

Braces for Adults

Braces are beneficial for just about anyone in terms of improving both their bite and their appearance. About the only person we would hesitate to put braces on would be a patient with periodontal (gum) disease that renders the underlying bone not healthy enough to support movement of the teeth.

Approximately 40% of our practice consists of treating adults. A lot of that is treatment with braces, but a lot more adults are now choosing clear aligner therapy such as Invisalign. Our practice, Blue Wave Orthodontics is in the Top 1% of Invisalign providers Worldwide, and that has substantially increased the number of adults we treat.

Within the past 15 years we have definitely seen a significant increase in the number of adults seeking orthodontic treatment. It's just become more and more socially desirable to have a really nice, attractive smile. That's usually the first thing someone notices when they look at you for the first time.

Over time, the stigma of having braces has been far outweighed by the stigma of not having a beautiful, straight smile. That's one reason more and more adults are getting treatment. We think the choice of having clear braces, replacing the metal braces that we used to use, has led to more people seeking out orthodontic cosmetic treatment. Plus, treatment times are faster now than before, because of the high-tech wires and brackets that we have available now, that move the teeth faster.

We do have to do some combination orthodontic treatment because sometimes, with some tooth movements, braces and wires will fix better, and some things aligners such as Invisalign will fix better. So, once in a while we may do some certain movements with braces and then complete the treatment with Invisalign. That way, instead of the patient having to have braces on for a year and a half to two years, they may only have braces on for three or four months, and then we can move them to treatment with Invisalign and finish in another 8-10 months.

The Development of Aligners

Treatment with aligners began in 1999. The new concept developed uses a succession, or progression, of clear aligners – aligners are essentially like clear retainers – that incrementally move your teeth more gently and easily without having to use braces. Invisalign is the main and original system developed. There are other aligner systems out there now, such as Clear Correct, but Invisalign still holds the original patent on the technology and is the aligner treatment of choice.

With Invisalign, you can go to an orthodontist, and they will scan your teeth with an optical/digital scanner to create an image. It takes about three minutes to take an image of the upper arch, and another three minutes to take an image of the lower arch.

Working on a computer from that image, sort of like working with a CAD – computer assisted design – program, the orthodontist is able to create a progressive series of clear trays called aligners to quickly move your teeth. This enables them to be incredibly precise, by modeling each tray based on the most recent scan, so that the orthodontist can create for the patient exactly the look, bite and smile that is desired.

Because the aligner trays are clear, there's no embarrassment for the patient in the way there once was with metal braces.

Treatment with Invisalign

Invisalign is a huge technological advance and quite frankly the first MAJOR paradigm shift to treat malocclusions since the specialty began in 1901. Invisalign enables us to treat patients over the age of 12 - basically anyone who has all their permanent teeth in – and get amazing results usually within a treatment time of just 12 months. Invisalign has enabled us to get great cosmetic results, often without doing extractions or surgery.

Treating the average patient with Invisalign takes about 12 months. The orthodontist uses an average of 48 lower and upper aligner models, designed from the 3D image scans. A UV light polymerizing resin is the main ingredient of the model, so we can take the Invisalign material and process it on each incrementally varied resin model. The "Smart Track" Align material is pressed down on the model, and a robotics program guides a laser to cut it. The freshly formed aligners are now tumbled with a bunch of ceramic beads to smooth the edges. They are then computer assisted labeled and bagged.

So now you have 48 sets of incrementally progressive aligners. The patient wears each set 22 hours a day for a week (or two) and then goes on to the next one. The aligners progressively move your teeth and you get a wonderful result at the end.

When the Invisalign treatment is complete, some patients may need some refinement, just tweaking the results a bit to get things even more ideal. The orthodontist does another scan and creates an additional three or four months' worth of trays that the patient wears to get really perfect results if needed or desired.

Also, patients will wear a retainer at night after completing the Invisalign treatment, to hold their results! Many opt for the Invisalign retainer called Vivera which is made like the aligners that move your teeth, only with Vivera they hold the final position!

And "voila", you are done and have gorgeous results with "look Ma, NO braces"!

Invisalign is an amazing technology, a total paradigm shift. It's almost like if you wanted to travel from New York to Los Angeles and the only available travel choices were train, bus, or car. In regard to orthodontics, Invisalign is like the paradigm shift that occurred when suddenly people were able to travel by airplane!

Advantages of Aligners

Probably about 95% of our adult patients use Invisalign. The only situations where we wouldn't use Invisalign are if the patient has an impacted tooth – a tooth stuck in their gums – or some other situation that necessitates surgery.

Some patients may need periodontal work done before they can use Invisalign. If you're going to move teeth, you've got to have a good, solid foundation for the teeth. You can't move teeth if the patient has significant periodontal or gum disease because there's not a strong enough foundation. Those patients would first need treatment by a periodontist who examines them to decide which teeth are good and which ones are poor or guarded. We would remove the poor teeth and the guarded ones need cleaning before you can do orthodontic treatment.

Aligners can offer several advantages over using braces. Braces can stick to your teeth and bother your lips. Also, braces can potentially damage the enamel coating on the teeth, especially with poor oral hygiene. Although that's not as big a problem now as it was when braces were always made of metal. Braces can pick up a little food debris where the bracket meets the tooth, and then bacteria can begin to cause decay.

What can happen if the patient doesn't brush well enough and the dentist doesn't catch it, when they take off the brackets, there are little white rings on their teeth, the beginnings of a cavity AKA decalcification. Potentially, that might mean having to get bonding or veneers after straightening the teeth. When you use aligner therapy, you don't have that problem.

With braces, you also still have the social stigma of wearing them, which bothers some patients, and more pain or discomfort than you have with aligners.

With Invisalign, you can just pop the aligners on and off, take them off for eating or for a date or other social engagement. They feel much more comfortable than braces, and they don't affect your speech. Plus, you don't have the problem that braces have of picking up plaque and bacteria. With aligners, you're changing the tray every week or two, so you regularly have a brand-new tray that's fresh and clean.

Having recommended aligners from the beginning, 1999 we have had many celebrities, beauty contestants, sports figures, musician, weather announcers and news broadcasters that wear them as prescribed, i.e. all the time, when performing and "on the air" with no issues at all!

Aligners are clean, they're healthy, and they look good. Most people cannot even tell when you have a clear aligner on. That's one of the reasons that so many adults absolutely love Invisalign treatment, because it doesn't show like braces do.

Cost of Orthodontic Treatments

As a general rule, the cost for treatment with braces ranges from about $3,000 to around $7,000, depending upon the type and length of treatment and what part of the world you live in. Patients who finance the treatment typically pay about $150 to $250 per month in payments, depending upon the dental practice's financing policies. Many practices, including ours, offer an in-house financing plan.

Dental insurance, depending on the company, usually covers part of the cost, but usually not all of it, which is why most orthodontists offer patients a financing or payment plan.

Aligners, depending upon the length of treatment, run in about the same price range, from around $3,000 up to about $7,500.

Our practice is Invisalign/Braces neutral, meaning we charge the same to get the malocclusion corrected. We do NOT surcharge for Invisalign.

The generally reduced orthodontic treatment times have made it easier for dentists to offer their patients financing, since obviously, the cost depends a lot on how many times, and for how long overall we need to see and treat the patient.

Effectiveness of Orthodontic Treatments

Orthodontics treatments are really one of the most effective cosmetic dental procedures. They can make a big difference in someone's life. We get a lot of satisfaction when we can do something like treat a child who's been teased about the appearance of their teeth, and watch the treatment help them blossom into an outgoing, self-confident kid. That's one of the most rewarding parts of our profession.

We also treat a lot of adults that choose to finally get their teeth fixed, and the most common thing they say is that they wish they'd done it sooner. Just like with treating children, we've treated a lot of adults and have satisfaction seeing how getting their teeth fixed with braces or aligners just completely changes their personality as far as their self-esteem, self-confidence, and just their overall satisfaction in life.

Most HR people involved with interviewing job candidates always note one's smile is the most significant part of the non-verbal interview, and that makes all the difference.

Here's the story of just one case we treated. *The patient was a female air force officer in her late 20s. She had what's referred to as a severe Class III – that's where the lower jaw is much more forward than the upper jaw. She also had a severe underbite, the lower front teeth being way out in the front of the upper front teeth.*

She could have easily been a candidate for jaw surgery, but she specifically said that she didn't want to have jaw surgery.

We decided to go with Invisalign, which we thought we could make work for her without needing surgery. We had to extract her two lower front teeth, but after 15 months of

Invisalign treatment, we had closed up that space where the two teeth were removed, her underbite vanished and we were basically able to get the same results as if she'd had jaw surgery.

She was absolutely thrilled, both with the awesome results we were able to get for her and for the fact that she didn't have to have jaw surgery. Her "before" and "after" pictures show just an amazing transformation in her looks, and she, herself, said that the Invisalign treatment changed her life.

The technological advances that we've made in orthodontics, the development of better braces and the introduction of the Invisalign technology, have made it easier for both children and adults to get fantastic results as far as transforming their smile into a real work of art. We urge anyone who has a problem with the alignment of their teeth or their bite to look into their options by seeing and talking with an orthodontist.

About Randy Feldman, DDS, MS

Bluewave Orthodontics
www.BlueWaveOrtho.com

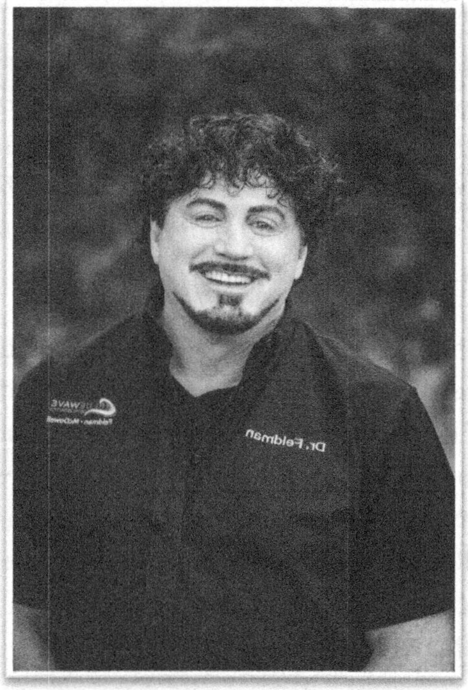

Dr. Randy Feldman received his BA in zoology from The Ohio State University, where he also obtained his DDS and MS in orthodontics. He is a Clinical Associate Professor in the Department of Pediatrics at USF College of Medicine. He also holds a patent for one of his contributions to the dental field, ceramic brackets. His passion is pediatric orthodontics, and for more than 30 years, he has been helping children obtain the smiles that they deserve. His special focus is helping special needs children. He is the former President of the Make-A-Wish

Foundation, sits on the board of directors for Voices for Children, and serves as a Guardian Ad Litem to the Florida judicial system. He is also the President of More Health, Inc., a group that promotes health education for students in Pinellas and Hillsborough Counties, and established the Feldman Orthodontics Scholarship Program to help send local Bay area students to college.

Additionally, Dr. Feldman is an early adopter of the Invisalign technique (1999) and is not only in the Top 1% of providers Worldwide, but he has also treated over 3,000 patients with this new innovative orthodontic process.

Dr. Feldman is a member of the American Association of Orthodontics, American College of Dentists (Fellow), American Cleft Palate Association, American Orthodontic Society, International College of Orthodontists (Fellow), American Dental Association, Southeastern Society of Pediatric Dentistry, Southern Association of Orthodontists, Florida Dental Association, Hillsborough County Dental Association(Past President), Tampa Bay Academy of General Dentistry (Mastership) and Schulman Study Group, as well as many other professional and community organizations. A few of his awards include the Tampa Bay Business Journal Health Care Hero, Greater Tampa Chamber Business of the Year (1997), Lifetime Achievement Award by the Hillsborough County Dental Association in 2011 and chosen as the Tampa Bay Lightning Community Hero in 2015.

The Consequences of Missing Teeth

"Doc, do I really need to replace that tooth?" This is a question that I, as a general dentist, often hear from someone who's faced with the loss of a tooth or who's been without one for several years—especially if it's a tooth that isn't really visible when the patient smiles or which is causing pain.

The simple answer is, "Yes, absolutely." Replacing a missing tooth is crucial not only to restore normal chewing and cosmetics but to the overall health of the entire body. God did not create us with spare teeth. Every tooth in our mouth serves a critical function and, if a tooth is lost, this can result in one or more consequences including significant nutritional insufficiencies as well as a predisposition to obesity, diabetes, coronary artery disease, and some forms of cancer.

Therefore, it's not only about replacing a missing tooth but about the overall health of the patient. Loss of a single tooth starts a domino effect that slowly but surely causes many serious problems as time goes by. Some of these changes are immediate and others take years, but all are predictable and inevitable.

In America today, more than 36 million people have lost all their natural teeth, and 120 million people in the U.S. are missing at least one tooth. These numbers are expected to grow in the next two decades.

The Causes of Tooth Loss

Before we talk in detail about replacing missing teeth and why it's so important to do this, it's imperative to understand the causes of tooth loss. Tooth loss results from decay, gum disease, injury, illness, or, simply, wear.

In my practice, I see patients who've had one or more missing teeth for a long time. Even though it's a medically necessity, for whatever reason, their previous dentist didn't stress the need for replacement. No one has ever explained to these patients the need to restore a properly balanced bite for overall health.

On the other end of a spectrum, patients come to my office with a broken tooth that can't be saved due to decay or injury, or they have a loose tooth caused by periodontal disease in which the supporting bone is lost. All of these scenarios lead to the same discussion about the need to replace a missing or soon-to-be-missing tooth or teeth.

If a patient is missing all their teeth, this is known as edentulism. Edentulism affects our most vulnerable populations—the aging and the economically disadvantaged. In the geriatric population, about 23 million individuals are completely edentulous, and about 12 million are edentulous in either the upper or lower jaw.

Approximately 90% of people who've lost all their teeth have dentures. It's been projected that the number of partially edentulous patients will continue to increase in the next 15 years to more than 200 million individuals. Partial edentulism affects a majority of adult Americans.

Understanding the Consequences of Missing Teeth

I treat people with missing teeth of all ages and from all walks of life. It may be a parent who dedicated themselves to their kids' health first and is now ready to address their own dental issues. It could be a professional who's competing in a corporate environment and needs a perfect smile. It may be a young person who never had the means to replace missing teeth and now finally has a job that offers dental insurance. Sometimes, it's a middle-aged woman who realizes that living without all her teeth is affecting her health. All these patients who are living with the consequences of tooth loss require proper professional guidance to decide on the best treatment option for their particular case.

This brings me to the biggest challenge I have as a practitioner: trying to educate a patient that doesn't go to the dentist regularly but is faced with immediate tooth loss and the need to replace that tooth or teeth. A typical example of this is a patient who had several, single-tooth extractions over the years and is used to having missing teeth. Because of the gradual, years' long deterioration, that patient is unaware of how these missing teeth are affecting not only their oral but overall health. He or she just accepts the situation as "normal." Good communication, establishing trust, and paying careful attention to the needs of these patients is key to guiding them toward restoring proper function and overall health.

The Effects of Missing Teeth on Health

The effects of missing teeth, other than the obvious aesthetics, are somewhat subtle and often don't create immediate problems. First, let's discuss the social consequences. If someone has missing teeth that are visible when they smile, that person often has low self-esteem and self-confidence. They cover their mouth when smiling, try to cover their teeth with the lips, or, worse yet, don't smile. We realize missing teeth affect how others regard us in both personal and professional situations and act accordingly when interacting with others. I regularly see patients who have developed certain habits in an attempt to cover up missing teeth that are visible when they speak or smile.

The physical effects of missing teeth are several and include:

Bone loss. As soon as a tooth is extracted or lost, the bone that held it in place starts filling in the resulting extraction socket, but the bone never reaches the same vertical or horizontal volume as when the tooth was still there. This is an important consideration to keep in mind, especially if the treatment plan is to restore the missing tooth with a dental implant. We usually graft the extraction site with particle bone from a cadaver. This grafted bone is absorbed and replaces the patient's own bone within three months as part of body's natural body healing process.

Bite shift. The spread of the same masticatory, or chewing, force over fewer teeth subjects all the remaining teeth to fracture, wear, and movement. Our chewing muscles don't become weaker just because we lose a tooth, but now we're chewing with fewer teeth using the same force as before the tooth loss.

Migration or movement of adjacent teeth and teeth in the opposing arch. When a tooth is missing, the adjacent teeth no longer have anything to hold them in place or to stop the teeth in the opposing arch from erupting (extending upward or downward from the gum line). Muscles, gravity, and chewing act upon the remaining teeth and cause movement of the adjacent or opposing teeth almost immediately. I've seen noticeable changes in just a few weeks.

Injury to intraoral tissues. This is caused by food particles that are no longer deflected and are larger in size because there are less teeth to chew. Tooth shape is not accidental. Each contour, groove, and cusp plays a crucial role. One of the main functions of a tooth is to deflect food debris from the most vulnerable areas of the gum. When the tooth is no longer there, that protection is gone, and soft tissues suffer the blunt forces of food particles hitting them. In addition, when a tooth is removed, the underlying bone resorbs (diminishes in volume) both vertically and horizontally, which, over time, because there is no tooth to deflect particles, will result in the trapping, or impaction, of food.

"Sinking in" of the cheeks. The outward appearance of our lower jaw is partially determined by all teeth being present in the arch. If one or more teeth are missing, the cheeks sink in, and the tongue will fill those spaces where the teeth were as well. When teeth are lost, especially in the back of the mouth, the outside appearance of the cheeks develops a sunken-in look.

Collapsed vertical dimension of the face and creases at the corners of the mouth. When there are no teeth in the back to chew with or have a what's known as a vertical stop. When the back teeth are missing, the whole face collapses as the chin comes closer to the nose. Creases at the corners of the mouth are a dead giveaway of a collapsed posterior bite. Do you remember the face of the old witch from classical children books and cartoons? Well, that's the collapsed vertical dimension of the face that I'm describing here.

Delayed effects of missing teeth include:

Super-eruption of the opposing tooth or teeth. As time goes by, the tooth on the opposing arch to the tooth that's been lost—especially if it's a tooth in the upper jaw—will just keep erupting. I often see cases in which the tooth touches the opposing gum area on the opposite arch if a tooth is missing and hasn't been replaced.

Periodontal disease results in bone loss that leads to increased tooth mobility and possible additional tooth loss. As a tooth continues to super-erupt, it moves out of the bone socket. This creates inflammation of the gum and bone loss around the adjacent—and otherwise healthy—teeth. Teeth don't only erupt in a vertical direction. When a tooth is missing, an adjacent tooth will begin to lean. This creates a food trap, which is followed by chronic inflammation and bleeding that causes bone loss. This is known as a periodontal pocket. Once the bone is lost, it can never be replaced, and the support of the tooth is weakened. This ultimately results in the loss of that tooth as well. This domino effect must be stopped as soon as possible.

Continued and pronounced tooth migration leading to food traps and decay in adjacent teeth. As time goes by, adjacent and otherwise healthy teeth surrounding the area where the tooth is missing continue to lean into the unoccupied space. This creates food traps between the teeth, making it difficult if not impossible to maintain good oral health, which causes decay. The same thing can happen in the opposing arch—the tooth super-erupts, creating food traps among adjacent teeth. In addition, a super-erupted tooth exposes a softer tooth layer, which is prone to decay.

Temporomandibular joint (TMJ) disease or temporomandibular disorder (TMD). The musculature of our head and neck are affected by the smallest of changes. Single or multiple missing teeth can cause pain in the joint/jaw and elsewhere in the head and neck. Once a patient develops TMJ pain due to tooth loss, it's a long road back to health that involves many months and, in some cases, years of phased treatment to correct the problem. In some severe cases, surgery is necessary to relieve chronic TMJ pain.

Significant nutritional changes are observed in patients who are completely or partially edentulous (if they have a large number of missing teeth). If people have missing teeth, it makes it difficult to chew certain foods that are high in vitamins, minerals, and other nutrients. These foods include fruits, raw vegetables, nuts, and meat. The changes resulting from nutritional deficits have been shown to lead to obesity, coronary artery disease, diabetes, and even some forms of cancer.

Options for Treating Missing Teeth

Modern dentistry has many options to restore missing teeth and prevent the unwanted consequences of tooth loss. Before we get into restorative options, it's necessary to discuss socket (bone) preservation.

If a patient is faced with immediate tooth loss or an extraction, preserving as much of the supporting jawbone as possible is crucial for the future success of any restoration. Bone preservation is accomplished by performing the most nontraumatic tooth removal possible followed by a bone graft. For optimal results, a dentist must have a good extraction technique to preserve as much bone as possible.

What are your options for missing teeth?

Do Nothing

Of course, one response to a situation of missing teeth is to do nothing, but that's not a good one for the reasons we've discussed above—resultant bone loss, bite shift, migration of adjacent teeth, super-eruption, etc. Often patients feel that replacing a tooth that isn't visible when they smile is a waste of money, but, as discussed, not replacing a tooth will lead to many serious problems.

Fixed Permanent Bridges

A bridge is a permanently cemented dental appliance that is used to replace one or more missing teeth. In case of a single missing tooth, the teeth on either side of that missing tooth are carefully shaped and used as anchors to support a row of three, connected crowns, known as units—one to fill in the gap where the tooth is missing and two on the adjacent teeth.

For more than one missing tooth, a bridge can be extended to replace several missing teeth. In these cases, where many teeth are missing but there are critically located teeth remaining, we can install an extended fixed bridge. It can be of any length and extend as much as needed to correct the missing-teeth problem. Bridges of five, six, or eight units can be used. In extreme cases, a bridge can extend from the rear molar on one side of the jaw to the rear molar on the other side—10 to 14 units in a single appliance. This type of fixed bridge is called a roundhouse. A bridge could replace every tooth in the mouth depending on where the abutment teeth—the teeth that hold the bridge in place—are located and what shape they're in.

For lost-tooth replacement, a bridge was the recommended option for many years. One reason was that, up until five or 10 years ago, insurance companies would cover a bridge but not an implant.

Because placement of a bridge uses the adjacent teeth on either side to hold the replacement tooth in place, this means that two (in most cases) perfectly healthy teeth must be trimmed down to accommodate the crown.

Another downside of a bridge is that it can cause nerve irritation that may necessitate a root canal. A root canal is microsurgery, and each root canal is different. A root canal can create issues with lateral or accessory canals, so it's better to never touch a virgin tooth.

Bridges can also create difficult-to-clean areas, leading to future decay, and they don't address the bone-loss issue. In addition, they have a high failure rate over time, because we lose gum and bone tissue as we age, and this creates spaces in the bridge that can become susceptible to decay.

Considerations for deciding which type of bridge is best are based on the individual clinical situation, and the primary deciding factor is where the remaining supporting teeth are in relation to the missing ones.

A cemented, permanent bridge is the proper restoration of choice in some cases. However, today, with the availability of implants, I believe a bridge is an inferior option for tooth replacement. I feel recommending a bridge is a disservice to my patients, because it means I'm taking a single-tooth problem and making it a multi-tooth problem. Why involve other teeth when we can focus all our efforts and treatment on the one tooth that's missing? Why look for a more destructive solution when a simple, more predictable, and similarly priced one is available? I discuss this in detail below.

Dentures

A denture is a removable dental appliance used to replace a section of missing teeth (partial denture) or all the missing teeth on an upper or lower jaw (full denture). Dentures are, essentially, plastic trays with teeth attached that sit over the gums. Dentures offer the advantage of being a more affordable option than bridges or implants.

Dentures can solve cosmetic and bite-alignment issues, but they don't solve the problem of bone loss. As a result, patients need to have a new denture made every few years. The ongoing, gradual bone loss causes the jaw to shrink and, eventually, the dentures no longer fit.

Another problem with dentures is that they're prone to shift and move. Upper dentures, which cover the roof of the mouth, can cause a loss of the sense of taste. Some people are unable to tolerate upper dentures, because they can stimulate the gag reflex if the denture plate extends to the back of the palate.

• *Removable Partial Dentures*

In the case of multiple missing teeth, a removable partial denture (RPD) is the most cost-effective option. RPD restores function well and is economical. Unlike implants and bridges, an RPD must be removed overnight and stored in a cleaning solution. It can also rub on gum tissue and cause anchoring teeth to become mobile, break, and, ultimately, be lost.

• *Full Dentures*

For a patient with no teeth on the upper or lower jaw or both, the most cost-effective option is a full denture (FD). For the upper jaw, these are easy to make fit and stay in place because of suction, but, on the lower jaw, maintaining the stability of a full denture during chewing is a difficult proposition. There's minimal suction, and the tongue, lips, and cheeks act on the denture and can dislodge it.

Also, because of changes in the jawbone and gum tissue, dentures often need to be remade every five years. When people wear the same dentures for a long time, they get comfortable with them. But the jawbone constantly remodels. As the matter of fact, all bones in our body remodel. There's no bone tissue in our body that's over 11 years old. So, the result of wearing any removable denture over five years is that the bone it's sitting on is no longer same shape, size, or density as when the denture was made. The jawbone tissue is resorbed, vertical dimension is lost, and it looks like the person has no teeth. This gives an appearance of aging that's far beyond the actual chronological age of the patient. A new denture will make any patient appear younger. TMJ issues can arise as well from the gradual grinding down of the dentures and resorption of the bone.

Implants

Dental implants are the only treatment for a missing tooth that actually focuses on restoring that tooth and doesn't involve any other teeth or structures. It's also the only treatment that permanently addresses bone loss. Because of their many benefits—including being the most conservative option—implants have become the standard of care for replacing missing teeth. Whenever possible, an implant is my treatment of choice. I use implants to I restore missing teeth in members of my family, and they're my first recommendation for my patients as well.

A dental implant is a titanium screw that replaces the root of a missing tooth. During a simple, 15-minute, surgical procedure, the implant is installed in the space where the tooth is missing. In most cases, I work through a small, round opening in the gum, which means minimal pain, no stitches, and, usually, no post-op bleeding. Over the three months following surgery, the implant is integrated into the jawbone. Once the integration is complete, a simple impression is taken, and a specially trained laboratory technician fabricates the crown to be placed over the implant, which is cemented in place. This implant-supported crown has the same look and function as the natural tooth it replaced.

An implant is, by far, the most conservative and predictable method to restore a single missing tooth. An implant prevents bone loss by creating what's called "loading" on the bone, which is accomplished when the tooth opposing the missing tooth encounters solid resistance all the way through to the bone.

One reason an implant is preferable to a fixed bridge is there's no need to trim the healthy teeth adjacent to the gap where the tooth was. The cost of a single implant is the same or even less than that of a bridge, and the long-term success is greater, making it a better value.

Implants can last a lifetime. In my opinion, the main barrier to opting for implants is the health history and social habits of the patient. Implants are not a good option for smokers, people with insulin-dependent diabetes, or a history of certain drug use. Beyond those considerations, it's absolutely the best solution and the only one I recommend to patients seeking the best possible result. Why? Implant failure rate is almost zero. In addition, nothing is touched or disturbed in the mouth other than the area of the tooth that's being replaced. Any other option can cause future problems elsewhere in the mouth—to adjacent teeth or gums or the jawbone. I prefer to keep the treatment as localized as possible.

One of my patients is a 45-year-old man who is a tech for Verizon. He works outside most of the time. He has a high decay rate and, as the result, almost every tooth in his mouth has had a root canal done. When teeth are treated with root canals, they become brittle and weak, so any excessive pressure can cause these teeth to crack. One day, this patient was digging a trench, clenched his jaw too hard, and one of his upper teeth that had been treated with a root canal broke.

Obviously, this had to be addressed ASAP. We got him in right away on an emergency basis, and I evaluated the problem. Because all his other teeth were undamaged—although they had been treated with root canals and crowned—we decided to leave them undisturbed and restore the broken tooth with an implant.

During that first emergency visit, I extracted the remaining root fragment, grafted the socket to preserve the bone volume, and fabricated a removable, one-tooth denture called a flipper. A flipper isn't meant for chewing and serves two purposes. One is to hold the space to prevent tooth migration, and the second is cosmetic—allowing the patient to go out in public and to work. After three months, I placed an implant into the space of the missing tooth, and the patient continued wearing the flipper for an additional three months as the implant was integrated into the bone. After three months, an impression was taken and sent to the lab, which fabricated a crown to fit over the implant. This crown looks and functions the same as the tooth it replaced—and, because of the extreme strength of the implant, I would argue it's even better. This restoration involved no other teeth, and the patient is extremely happy with the results. This case addressed aesthetics as well as function.

As I think of the benefits that dental implants offer, another case comes to mind. My mother was a dentist in New York and, among many of her patients, she had one lady who absolutely loved her. After my mother retired, this woman didn't go to the dentist for almost 20 years. She finally came to me, but, by that time, she had many broken and missing teeth. Her partial denture no longer fit her mouth, and she had severe jawbone resorption.

She wanted to restore her mouth so she could chew properly again, and she wanted to avoid dentures. Her front four teeth were cosmetically okay, but she didn't really care about cosmetics that much. Her primary concern was having permanent back teeth in her upper jaw so she could chew well.

A Cone Beam Computed Tomography (CBCT) scan showed there just might be enough bone for implants, which would give her what she wanted. This was an extremely challenging situation. I'd have to "thread the needle" perfectly to place the six implants in a way that would be successful. I decided that guided-implant placement was the best option. A special surgical guide was milled on a 3D printer using the information from the CBCT scan. This guide was used to place the implants with extreme precision and proper angulation.

In addition to implants, she needed to have bone grafts in her sinuses to further stabilize the implants and, ultimately, the replacement teeth. The main challenge was that, over the years, her bone had resorbed to such an extent that the implants needed to be placed at extreme angles. The ultimate goal of placing teeth in proper orientation guided every design decision in this case including during implant-placement surgery. Meticulous planning and understanding of the end goal were essential so the result she was looking for could be achieved.

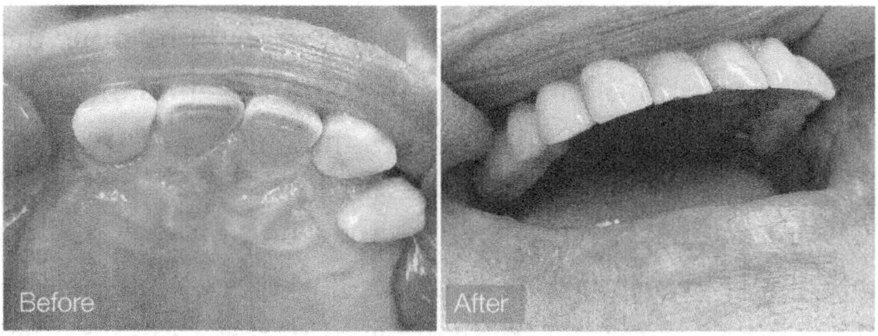

Placing two implant-supported bridges

In the end, all challenges were met, and she loved the results. Even though we started with a severe bone loss situation, we were able to overcome it and make the patient happy. She can chew well on both sides of her mouth, and her remaining front teeth weren't touched. I'm especially pleased with the results of this surgery. Even though this patient waited too long and had severe bone loss, we were able to treat her successfully with implants.

Hybrid Options

• *Implant-supported Dentures*

In my many years of practice, I've seen only a handful of patients who are completely satisfied with their lower FD (full dentures). Luckily, modern dentistry has an answer. We can place implants with male attachments that fit into female receivers in the base of the FD to keep it tightly in place.

The number of implants is determined by the anatomy of the remaining jawbone and surrounding structures such sinuses, nerves, and blood vessels—and, of course, the patient's budget. A lower FD can be stabilized by as few as two and as many as six implants. The remaining bone dictates the position, length, and the width of implants to be placed and, therefore, determines the number.

For a patient with no teeth in their bottom jaw, the best solution is to install four implants into the jawbone to stabilize it and, after the implants heal in three months, ball attachments are installed. A denture is made on which there are four sockets on the underside. These are basically rubber gaskets that go over the metal balls on top of the implants and click into place. The denture is removed at night like ordinary dentures.

This method stabilizes the denture better than anything I've ever seen and preserves the bone around the implants. This approach, which is called an implant-supported overdenture, is the least expensive and most economical approach to restore almost full function. The same process can be used for the upper jaw.

• *Implant-supported Fixed Bridge*

The option that ensures the best quality of life for a patient with an edentulous arch is an implant-supported fixed bridge. This bridge is attached to eight to 10 implants, can be made in one or more sections, is permanent, and looks and feels almost like the patient's original healthy teeth. This option is available to anyone with sufficient remaining jawbone.

These restorations have transformed the lives of my patients. For example, one of my patients is an older woman who was tired of her ill-fitting dentures. She also had broken-down teeth under permanent bridges and crowns. Her bite was inadequate, and she was very frustrated with this situation. She felt the time had come to address her dental problems once and for all.

When she came in, she was reluctant to smile. When speaking, she would try to hold her lips tight and even put her hand over her mouth. She was embarrassed by how much her oral health had deteriorated. I didn't judge her but rather listened carefully, examined her mouth, and put her mind at ease. Her case involved several steps but wasn't complicated. She just needed someone to understand and help her. She didn't need a CBCT scan, because, with my experience, I was able to look at her jaw and say, "No problem. We can do this for you."

She had enough bone that I could do a full, permanently cemented, implant-supported bridge on her top jaw and an overdenture retained by four implants on the bottom jaw. I explained the steps involved in the treatment, and she appreciated being fully informed. This relaxed her to the point where she was even looking forward to her appointments.

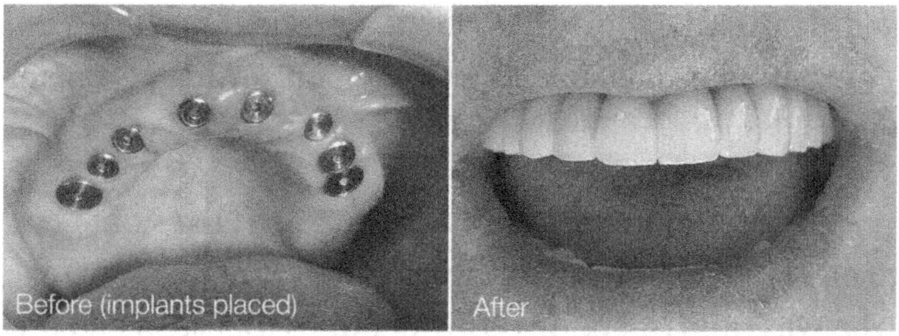

Placing an implant-supported bridge

This case involved me extracting her remaining decayed teeth and root fragments, bone grafting the extraction sockets, fabricating upper and lower full dentures for her to wear while the surgical sites healed, and then, three months later, placing eight implants on the top and four on the bottom. Three months after the implants were placed, the implant-supported restorations were fabricated —for the top, a permanently cemented, 10-unit bridge and, for the bottom, a denture retained by four, strategically placed implants. She was thrilled with the results and said having implants changed her life completely. She's learning how to smile all over again!

Determining the Best Option for Restoring Missing Teeth

Understanding the patient's needs, goals, and expectations along with careful treatment planning is crucial in determining the long-term success of tooth replacement options. The assessment should include available diagnostic modalities such as CBCT, 3D-milled precision surgical guides, and diagnostic casts and wax-ups. A complete medical and dental history is critical as well.

One concern that patients have is the amount of pain involved in the various treatment options. I can safely say that, in my practice, implant surgery is the least painful of all major dental procedures. Over 90% of my patients report little to no discomfort. Some don't even take over-the-counter analgesics like Advil or Tylenol following the procedure.

The good news is that modern dentistry performed by a competent, experienced practitioner offers many great options for replacement of missing teeth—whether it be one, several, or all, recently extracted or missing for decades.

The most important decision you can make about your treatment is to find a compassionate, qualified, experienced, well-trained, conscientious, knowledgeable, dental professional who will listen and understand all your concerns and goals. There's no single way to treat any one case, so good communication and honest discussion with your dentist is crucial for the best long-lasting results.

About Alexander Rockwell, DMD

Rockwell Dentistry
www.RockwellDentistry.com

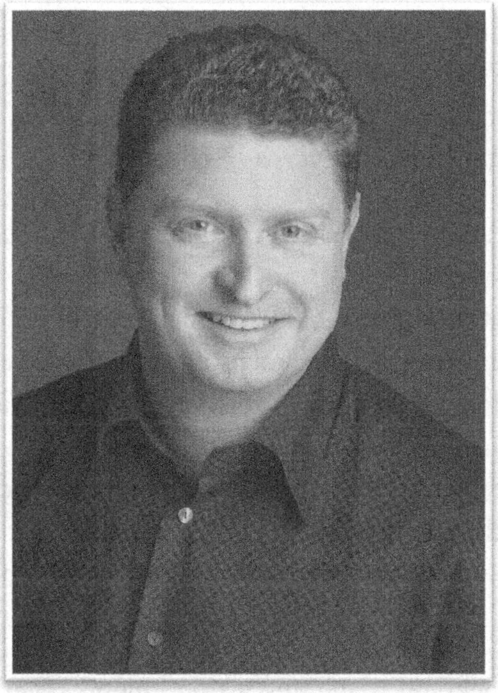

Originally from Kiev, Ukraine, Dr. Alexander Rockwell immigrated to the United States with his parents when he was 12 years old. By age 15, he was already working as an assistant in his mother's dental practice, and he knew he wanted to follow in her footsteps. Today, he and his wife, Dr. Dawn Rockwell, provide comprehensive dental care to patients in Middletown and Hamilton, New Jersey, at Rockwell Dentistry. Doctors Alex and Dawn are looking forward to having their twin children, Eric and Natasha, who are in dental school now, join them.

Dr. Rockwell attended Brooklyn College in New York City and then earned his doctorate in dental medicine from Fairleigh Dickinson University in Teaneck, New Jersey. After dental school, Dr. Rockwell studied and gained experience in oral surgery, and endodontics. He also pursued advanced training in periodontics, implantology, and acute care. In addition to his private practice, Dr. Rockwell teaches at Temple University School of Dentistry.

As an attending doctor at Monmouth Medical Center's dental clinic in Long Branch, New Jersey, Dr. Rockwell provided training and taught clinical dentistry to the residents in the hospital's dental program. Today, he regularly participates in advanced courses, seminars, and study groups that address unique areas of dental care. He wants to ensure that every patient in his practice encounters a highly skilled, proficient, dental professional at the top of his game when it comes to providing state-of-the-art dental care.

Dr. Rockwell maintains affiliations in several professional organizations including the American Dental Association, American Academy of Implant Dentistry, and American Academy of Cosmetic Dentistry.

Filling the Gaps with Dental Implants

What is a Dental Implant?

In the simplest terms, dental implants serve as replacement tooth roots that provide a strong foundation for fixed (non-removeable) replacement teeth (crowns) that match the patient's natural teeth and provide a permanent solution for missing teeth. The basis for modern dental implants is a biologic process called osseointegration (which we'll talk about shortly). Osseointegration means that the material used in the implant—usually titanium— fuses with the jawbone.

Dental implants have many advantages over dentures, bridges, or other forms of tooth replacements because they look like natural teeth, improve chewing and speech (they don't slip like poor-fitting dentures do), and enhance the patient's self-esteem by providing a permanent, natural-looking smile.

Here's an example of how implants changed the life of one of my patients. This young lady was a 22-year-old college student who was born without lateral incisors, which are the teeth on either side of the two front teeth. The lack of these lateral incisors left gaps, and she was wearing a removable prosthesis. She'd been told she didn't have enough bone to place implants.

We told her we could do bone grafting to increase the amount of bone, and then place implants. We did the bone grafting, placed the implants, and installed crowns. Once she had the implants, she was no longer worried that her removable prosthesis might fall out when she was eating or embarrassed that people would notice these weren't her real teeth. Before we placed the implants and crowns, she had a little bit of a lisp when she talked that was caused by the ill-fitting prosthesis. Once she had the implants, her lisp went away entirely.

Those implants changed her life. Before we did anything, whenever she smiled, she tried to force her upper lip down over her top teeth in the hope that nobody could see that she had a prosthesis. Now when she smiles, it's a bigger, wider, happier smile.

The Implant is Just the Beginning

When people hear the word "implant," they often think that once they receive the implant, they're done. There are three components to an implant. There's the implant itself, which is the structure that goes into the bone—in other words, a replacement for the root of the tooth. there's what's called the abutment, which is a piece that's secured to the inside of the implant to provide support for the crown. The third piece, the crown, is the part of the tooth that's visible inside the mouth.

The implant is placed by an oral surgeon. After the healing period, the patient returns to the oral surgeon, who adds the abutment and places a temporary crown on that. The patient then goes to their general dentist to have impressions made and the final crown created. The crown is done like any other crown, except we make sure the margin is as flush as possible with the abutment, meaning there's no gap between the crown and the abutment. This can be done with greater accuracy using implants. We can copy the abutment exactly, so the crown usually fits very well. The abutment is the middle piece between the implant and the crown, and it supports the crown. The abutment can be made of many different materials—titanium, porcelain, or various kinds of ceramics. When aesthetics is a consideration, a porcelain or ceramic abutment is often used, because it looks more like the natural tooth color.

For the posterior teeth, we can use a titanium abutment and a porcelain fused to metal crown. This would give you a replacement tooth that is very strong and still provides an aesthetically pleasing outcome. The extra strength is important, because we do most of our chewing using our back teeth, our molars. For the front teeth, we often do a zirconia abutment, which is pressed porcelain, because it looks like the natural teeth and creates a natural-looking smile. The biting force on the front teeth is much less than it is in the posterior teeth.

Patients need to be sure their dentist is aware of all the different materials that can be used for implants so they can make the best selection for the situation.

Different Types of Implants and Leading Implant Manufacturers

Many people don't realize that dental implants have been around for years. The first modern dental implants, which resemble the implants we use today, were developed, manufactured, and used in the 1970s and 1980s by a company called Brånemark. This company is named after the Swedish orthopedic surgeon, Per-Ingvar Brånemark, who created the first dental implant in 1952. These implants were first placed in patients in 1965. The Brånemark company was the first to design and manufacture successful dental implants to replace teeth. There were dental implants before that, but they didn't have as high a success rate as the Brånemark root-formed implant.

There are different types of implants and several companies that make them. These implants are similar to one another, but they have slightly different characteristics. Most brands contain titanium, which is what the original implants were made of. Zirconia is another material that's used, but I don't do zirconia implants because there isn't enough research available on them, especially in terms of how long they last. Also, instead of there being three components to the implant, in the zirconia product, the implant and the abutment are one piece, which can make it harder to install the crown on top in the exact position desired.

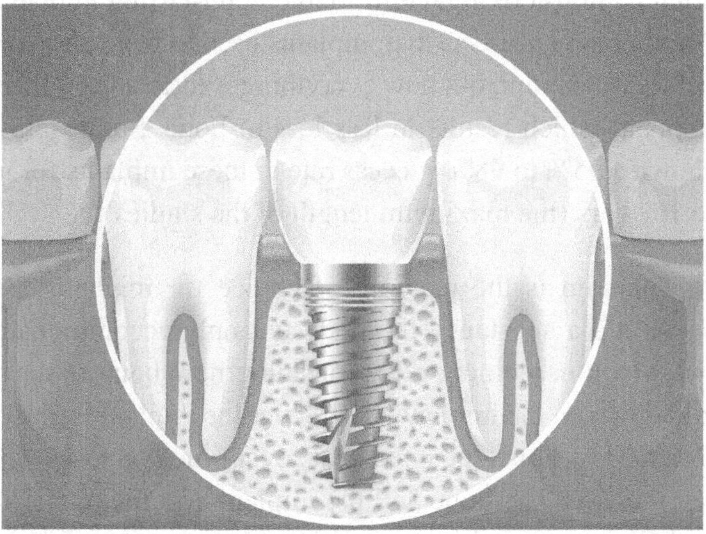

The largest manufacturers of implants in the United States are Zimmer Biomet 3i, BioHorizons, Nobel Biocare, Straumann, and Astra Tech. These companies have longevity, and their implants have been shown to last a long time.

Recent Improvements to Dental Implants

Many technical improvements have been made in implants over the past 70 years. Before the Brånemark implant, there were large dental implants and something called blade implants, which were placed between the soft tissue and the bone. These were durable, but when they failed, they often destroyed the bone.

Then dental implants became smaller and looked like the root of a tooth, which was a major step forward in creating natural-looking, comfortable, long-lasting implants. Another advance was that implants used to have an external fixation point, but now everything is internal inside the implant, which results in less loss of bone. Studies have shown a 95% to 98% success rate in these implants for up to 10 years (the maximum length of the studies).

Titanium is the material of choice for implants, because it's a substance the body not only accommodates but which osseointegrates—meaning new bone tissue is laid down on the implant itself. After the implant is placed into the jaw bone, the bone heals over time and fuses with the implant. The bone and the implant become one. This is the key to why dental implants today are so successful. Older implants, like the blade implant, never actually osseointegrated, so no fusion occurred.

Who's a Good Candidate for Implants?

I recommend dental implants for any patient who's missing teeth. Any missing tooth can be replaced with a dental implant if there's sufficient bone to place it. For a patient that's missing multiple teeth, we use an implant-supported bridge. For a single missing tooth, we replace that with a single implant. If a patient is missing all their teeth, implants can be used to replace all of their teeth.

There are different ways of replacing all the teeth with implants. Previously, we replaced every tooth with an implant or every other tooth with an implant using a bridge, but now we can replace the teeth with fewer implants and still create a strong enough foundation to hold a structure on top that replaces all the missing teeth. We angle the implants in a way that allows us to increase the number or size of the teeth that can be placed onto fewer implants. That way, we save the extra cost of more implants, and there are fewer complications and a higher rate of success.

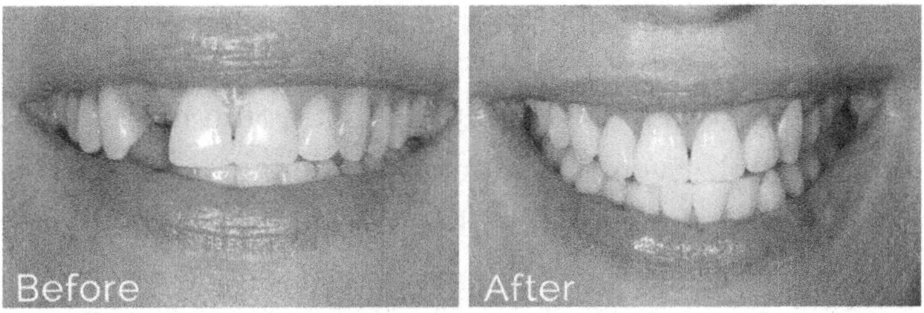

Single implant placement

WHO ISN'T A GOOD CANDIDATE FOR IMPLANTS?

We don't recommend implants for smokers, but they can be done for smokers if they agree to stop smoking prior to placing the implants and for a period of time after placing the implants. The nicotine in tobacco inhibits the healing potential of the bone. If a patient is a smoker, instead of a 98% success rate with the implant procedure, it will be more like a 75% success rate.

There are also certain medical conditions that make a patient more susceptible to infection, although we can usually accommodate this as well. Prior to placing implants, the patient should work with their general dentist to make sure any other problems in the mouth are taken care of—such as gum disease or cavities—because we don't want those to cause an infection in the implant.

The one big contraindication is not having enough bone structure to place the implants, which requires bone grafting by an oral surgeon before the implant can be placed.

Although it's rare, a person can have an allergy to titanium and therefore not be a candidate for dental implants.

There are very few conditions that would make dental implants fail. Even if a patient has a bone condition like osteoporosis, they could still be a candidate for implants. However, certain medications used to treat osteoporosis—specifically, bisphosphonates—can cause problems with the healing of the jaw bone. If a patient is on a bisphosphonate and undergoes an invasive dental procedure like an implant, this can lead to necrosis—death—of jaw-bone tissue. To determine if the surgery will be safe, it's necessary to evaluate when the patient started taking the medication and how long they've been on it. It's sometimes possible to have them stop taking the medication for a few months and then place the implant(s).

Cancer patients who've had metastases to their bones may be prescribed a bisphosphonate, often at higher doses than patients who have osteoporosis, so they may or may not be candidates for implants due to the risk of necrosis unless the patient is able to stop taking that drug for a few months prior to the implant procedure.

Young people require certain consideration when evaluating whether implants are appropriate. If a teenager suffers trauma, loses a tooth, and desires an implant, we need to be sure they've completed any orthodontic treatment, because it isn't possible to move the implant. All the teeth need to be aligned in the proper position before placing it. Secondly, it's necessary to be sure the young person isn't still growing, because, as they grow, that could shift the position of the implant.

The Implant Process

The implant time frame starts as soon as a tooth is lost or removed. The hole where the tooth used to be is surrounded by bone and gum tissue. As it starts to heal, this hole will fill in with bone and gum tissue and, as it does so, it starts to shrink.

If the bone tissue shrinks too much, there won't be sufficient bone to place the implant. That can happen as early as in the initial three months of the healing period. To prevent that shrinkage, a minimally invasive bone-graft procedure can be performed to place mineralized bone into the hole where the tooth used to be to inhibit shrinkage. This graft also acts as a scaffold for new bone growth.

If the bone graft isn't done and the area heals, the area will continue to shrink every year. Even if a bone graft is done, it's recommended that the implant be placed within one year, because shrinkage will still occur during that year. Why? Over a six- or eight-month period—the graft will be replaced by the patient's own natural bone. That natural bone, without being exposed to any of the usual forces of chewing and so on, will shrink. Without those biomechanical forces created by the presence of a tooth, there's nothing telling the bone to remodel, and it begins to shrink and resorb. So, it's important to reestablish those chewing forces to have a successful, long-term implant.

Therefore, it's important to do a bone graft or an implant as soon as possible after an extraction or other tooth-loss incident. There are certain situations in which an implant can be placed the same day the tooth is lost or removed. This requires a consult with an oral surgeon to be sure it's feasible.

After having the tooth removed and a bone graft placed the graft will need to heal for a 3 month period. Then the patient will return for a consultation to determine if the implant can be placed. The surgeon will most likely do what's called a cone-beam CT scan to get a 3D image, evaluate the area, and then see if there's enough bone to support the implant so it won't fail. If everything looks good and the patient is ready to proceed, we schedule a second visit to place the implant. Depending on the comfort level of the patient, the placement process might be done with local anesthesia or may require IV sedation. All the patient feels during this process is a little light pressure—no pain. After that, there's a follow-up visit one week later to check the healing process, and then we allow the area to heal for three months. During this three months the process of osseointegration will occur and the implant will fuse with the surrounding bone making it strong enough to support a crown.

The patient returns, and we take another X-ray or CT scan. If everything looks good, we start putting the abutment on top of the implant in preparation of installing the crown.

Another more precise way to place an implant is by using CT-guided surgery. We take the CT scan, put it into computer software, and then virtually place the implant into the bone on the CT scan. Once we have the implant exactly the way we want it, we send the scan through the software to a company that fabricates a guide. Using this guide allows the surgeon to place the implant to exactly where it was on the CT scan. If there's a potential problem, it's eliminated by the software and the guide, which assures the implant will be in the exact spot we want it to be. Basically, there's no room for human error.

How Long Do Dental Implants Last?

We have plenty of patients with implants that have lasted well beyond 10 years. It's possible for implants to last a lifetime if patients take care of them as they would their natural teeth. Although implants can't develop cavities, gum infections and bone infections can form around the implant.

It's very important that patients follow the instructions of their oral surgeon after the implant has been placed to make sure they're brushing, flossing, and caring for the implant properly, and they need to have their teeth cleaned every six months by their dental hygienist.

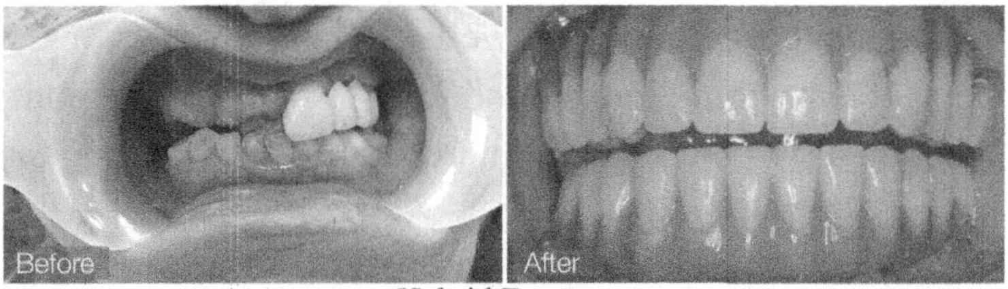

Hybrid Denture

Alternatives for Patients Who Aren't Candidates for Dental Implants

If a patient is only missing a single tooth or a few teeth, an alternative would be a bridge in which crowns are put on the teeth on either side of the space where the tooth is missing, and an artificial tooth is supported by the bridge.

The downside of bridges is that often there's nothing wrong with the teeth on either side of the lost tooth. To create a crown, it's necessary to shave the tooth down—removing healthy tooth structure—to put the crown on top of these teeth. With implants, it isn't necessary to do anything to the tooth next to the spot where the missing tooth was.

The other option is conventional dentures—either partial or full dentures. If a patient is missing all their teeth but is unable to have sufficient implants installed to support replacing all the teeth, they can do something called an overdenture, which uses fewer implants. A denture is made for the patient that's supported by the implants and the jaw bone. Both structures support the denture to make it stronger and more functional.

However, the problem with lower dentures is it's difficult to have suction that's as good as that on upper dentures, so they often don't fit well. The biggest complaint I hear about lower dentures is that they pop out frequently. If we're able to put denture clips into implants, this adds stability and prevents them from dislodging.

Part of the issue is that even though there's some pressure on the jaw bone from those dentures sitting on top of them, it's not the same degree of pressure as with a natural tooth or an implant. As a result, there's bone loss due to accelerated bone resorption, and then the dentures don't fit.

If implants are placed for aesthetic reasons rather than to improve chewing and create a better bite, there's no difference in how they're placed. Whether it's for function—such as in the posterior region of the mouth—or for aesthetics—because a tooth near the front is missing—the implant is always placed so it's aesthetically pleasing and functional. With a missing front tooth, the primary driving force behind getting the implant might be aesthetic, but we still want that implant to function properly so it will last.

How to Choose the Right Person to Do Dental Implants

Anyone with a dental license can place a dental implant. However, an oral surgeon has had four to six years of extra medical training as a resident, during which time they've placed thousands of implants and had training in other dental surgical procedures. Therefore, an oral surgeon has a lot more experience in placing implants, dealing with complications of this process, and in addressing issues relating to gum or bone problems.

Alternatively, a general dentist might take a few continuing-education classes here and there, but they have minimal experience in placing implants. Therefore, they are often learning as they go on you, the patient.

Usually, placing implants isn't that difficult, but, in those cases where complications arise, you're much better off with an oral surgeon. For example, there are certain anatomical considerations that must be taken into account when placing implants. There's a sinus cavity in the upper jaw above the back teeth. Many times, this sinus cavity is enlarged, which could result in insufficient thickness of the bone that causes the implant to puncture into the sinus cavity. Not only does this inhibit osseointegration, it carries a high risk of infection. Sometimes, there are procedures that make it possible to change the position of the sinus cavity and apply a bone graft that allows more room to place an implant.

In the lower jaw, there's a nerve that provides sensation to the lips, tongue, cheeks, gums, and chin. It's necessary to be very careful of this nerve, because even getting too close to it can cause damage and possible numbness to those areas. Choosing an experienced and skilled surgeon is vital in situations like that.

"Teeth in a Day"

One type of implant procedure is what's referred to as a hybrid denture. This is a solution for people who've lost all of their teeth in one arch or both (upper and lower arches). It provides total rehabilitation for patients with badly broken-down teeth, decayed teeth, or teeth compromised due to gum disease.

This process involves removing all the patient's teeth, replacing them with implants, and installing a hybrid denture on top of the implants. A hybrid denture isn't removable like usual dentures. It's screwed into the implants. It can be taken out by a dentist or an oral surgeon, but, for the most part, it's fixed into the mouth.

When we install hybrid dentures, we try to put at least four implants, which is the minimum. It's always better to put in an extra implant or two to provide better support. In the upper jaw, I prefer six, because it's a softer bone. I have no problem with five in the lower jaw, because it's a stronger, harder bone.

Hybrid Denture

Because this procedure requires at least four implants, it's often called "All-on-4" – "all" teeth supported "on four" implants. The term "teeth in a day" is also used to convey that the removing of the decayed or broken teeth and the placement of the hybrid denture can be done in one visit.

Normally, as I explained previously, a patient comes in for a consult, has a cone-beam CT scan done, and we provide them with an evaluation. The tooth-removal surgery is done on the next visit, the implant or implants could be a few months later if grafting is needed, and the crowns go on during the third visit, after a few more months, when the area is healed. This regular process can take a year. With "teeth in a day," the surgery, installation of implants, and application of the hybrid denture is done all in one visit, so the patient is never without teeth.

We recently saw a patient who'd struggled with her teeth throughout her life. This was a 58-year-old woman who had no access to dental care when she was growing up or for several decades thereafter. Now she was trying to take care of her teeth. However, her teeth were so far gone that she was having a lot of problems.

This patient had not only aesthetic issues but chewing problems. She didn't have a healthy diet, because she couldn't chew certain foods—in particular, vegetables—properly. By installing a hybrid denture, we gave her an aesthetic outcome that was very pleasing to her as well as a good functional outcome. As a result, her entire demeanor changed. She dressed and behaved differently. You could see she was happier.

ABOUT JAMES R. GREEN IV, DMD

Green Oral Surgery
www.OralSurgeonsTampa.com

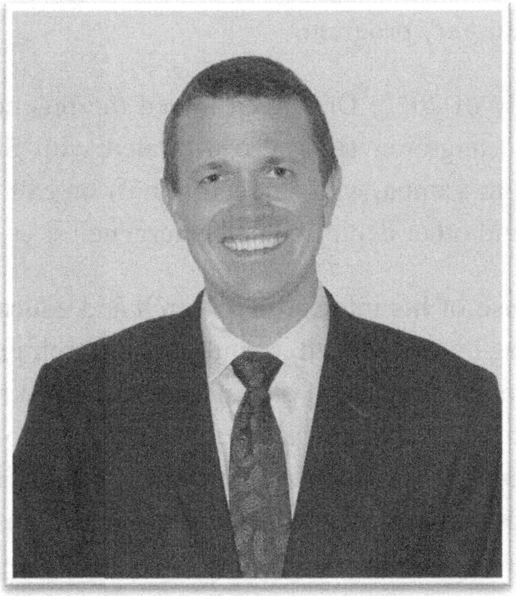

Dr. James R. Green is an oral and maxillofacial surgeon in Tampa, Florida. He was born and raised in Gainesville, Florida. Growing up in a family of "Gators" fans, he always desired to attend the University of Florida, which he did for his undergraduate and graduate studies. He received his Bachelor of Arts in Business Administration in 2003 and was accepted to attend the College of Dentistry. He obtained his Doctorate of Dental Medicine from the University of Florida in 2008.

Dr. Green completed his Oral and Maxillofacial Surgery and Anesthesia training at a Cornell affiliated hospital, The Brooklyn Hospital Center, in Brooklyn, NY. In his final year of residency, he acted as the chief resident of the oral surgery program.

In July of 2012, Dr. Green joined the practice of Dr. John P. Longmire. He's also affiliated with St. Joseph Hospital in Tampa, where he's routinely on call for facial trauma and other dental-related emergencies.

Because of his interest in research and education, Dr. Green has been involved in multiple research projects as well as presenting them at different scientific meetings. His research entails oral pathology, reconstruction, and facial trauma. He's also a contributing author in dental textbooks. He continues this interest in research and education through his involvement in the Hillsborough County Dental Research Clinic and the Tampa Dental Study Club.

Dr. Green is a member of multiple state and national associations in which he holds leadership positions. These associations include the American Association of Oral and Maxillofacial Surgeons, Florida Society of Oral and Maxillofacial Surgeons, American Dental Association, Florida Dental Association, and West Coast Dental Association. Dr. Green joined the Tampa Bay Lightning as the official oral surgeon for the 2014 season.

Dr. Green is supported by his wife, Lauren, and two children. He enjoys running and being with family and friends watching Florida Gator football games, but his favorite hobby is spending time with his children. Dr. Green and his wife are proud members of the Tampa community and enjoy giving back to local schools and charities whenever possible.

DR. CURTIS HAYES

Leading the Way with Digital Dentistry

The field of cosmetic dentistry is experiencing a major digital boom, thanks to all of the technological advances that are continually being made. Digital dentistry, in the simplest terms, refers to the use of digital, computerized technology in place of traditional techniques that have typically been used for dental procedures in the past. These new treatment methods and techniques are ever increasing in their scope and the opportunities they present to dentists and doctors around the world, helping to dramatically reduce or eliminate issues that may occur because of human error or inability to complete procedures and treatments with the most ideal results.

Dentistry is still partially a form of art, as well as a skill, so the human element is still absolutely necessary; human skill and vision is a predominant aspect of dentistry that allows patients to have the most stable and beautiful smiles. The digital aspect being brought in to dentistry is there to help dentists and doctors elevate their abilities and give their patients the smile of their dreams.

New Technology and Its Benefits

In my practice the biggest change in terms of digital dentistry is the addition of Cone Beam CT technology. This is a newer technology but one that is spreading rapidly throughout many dental offices. Within surgical care, this technology has become almost a standard of care. Cone Beam CT scanners differ from traditional CT scanners in that they capture images more quickly and use a much lower level of radiation.

Both Cone Beam CT scanners and traditional scanners fall into the tomography category of technology, however, the Cone Beam scanners are able to capture the information in one pass (less radiation) – versus a rotating x-ray tube used by traditional scanners which requires overlap of the slices. This new type of scan is a major improvement because it provides the dentist with a three-dimensional view of what's going on under the skin in the patient's mouth and jaw in an office setting. This enables the dentist to have a better understanding of exactly what they're dealing with when treating patients, especially when surgical or more invasive procedures are necessary.

Prior to the use of CT scans – especially the Cone Beam scanner - dentists and oral surgeons relied on traditional flat film, radiography - x-rays. These help to a point, but they don't provide a full image of the patient's condition. With only a two-dimensional image to work with dentists had to try to interpret – rather than precisely knowing – what was going on in a patient's mouth, jaw, and head. The major downside with flat films this is that while we often had correct interpretations of the condition, there were also times when we didn't. The Cone Beam scanner offers us the ability to be much more accurate in treating patients because it provides more clear and detailed information.

Here is a great example I just had when writing this chapter:

Karen is a 73 years old female patient who arrived to her general dentist with a complaint that her crown (that was placed by another dentist) keeps falling off. After careful inspection, the general dentist noted that there was not enough tooth structure to properly restore the tooth. He replaced the crown with temporary cement and sent her to my office.

Pre-operative x-ray given to me from her general dentist are shown on the left (note that the root canal). The patient was interested in getting an implant so we took a CT scan of the tooth to evaluate the bone quality (see that image on the right).

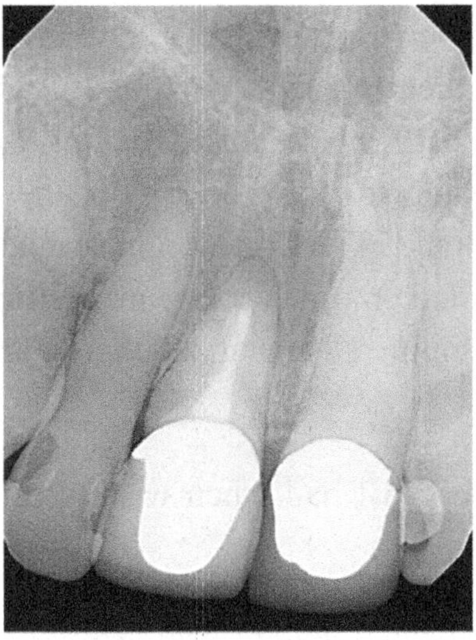

X-Ray

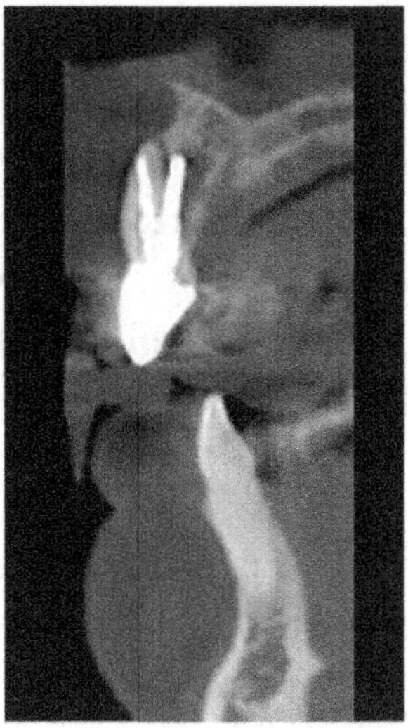

Cone Beam CT Scan

This CT scan shows that the root canal was completed correctly, but when it was restored with a post and core there were issues. The alternate view provided with this digital technology demonstrated that the post was placed outside the tooth and over time led to destruction of the bone behind the tooth. Without this bone an attempted immediate implant would have failed. Without the CBCT I would failed the patient and that is just another example of why I choose to be on the leading edge of digital dentistry.

More about Cone Beam Technology

I'd like to delve a little further into how Cone Beam technology works and how it helps me – and any dentist or surgeon using it – to better treat patients.

As I mentioned previously, using Cone Beam technology is an important part of helping dentists and oral surgeons plan and execute surgeries in the most effective way possible. Using the images provided by the scans, they can visualize the surgery and actually conduct a practice surgery on the computer. They are able to see things better such as the patient's bone density, tooth positions, and the patient's anatomy when it comes to things like nerve or sinus location, bone quality, and space needed for implants. Virtually doing the surgery before actually touching the patient, planning what needs to be done, as well as determining the best ways to accomplish these things ahead of time, makes it much easier to do the actual surgery in the best manner possible and get the best result for the patient.

Unfortunately, Cone Beam technology isn't yet a standard in every dentist's office. It's one of the newer technologies available. Fortunately, it is rapidly growing in use, especially among oral surgeons, orthodontists, endodontists, and periodontists.

Traditional Impressions

Before I can talk about digital impressions I think it's important to explain what traditional impressions are to help you compare and contrast the two. Prior to the creation of digital impressions, dentists were – and still are, in many offices – using alginate-or vinylpoly siloxane (big words that describe the type of materials used) impressions. Basically, these materials start as a gooey liquid and are put into a tray that is then inserted into the patient's mouth. The materials then begin to harden, making an impression of the patient's teeth. Before the materials dry entirely, the tray is removed from the patient's mouth and set out to become completely hard. Afterward, a stony material is then poured into the impression to create a solid, physical model of the patient's teeth.

There are considerable disadvantages to this method of creating impressions. Each of the materials used to create these impressions has different expansion and contraction rates, meaning they can shrink or expand. They are very sensitive to humidity and environmental temperatures. Any or all of those factors can affect how the model accuracy when compared to the patient's teeth ends up being.

Another one of the major disadvantages of the traditional impression method is how patients react to these impressions. Most don't like the sensation of the gooey material in their mouth, the size of the tray used to hold the material, and how difficult it can be to remove the tray once the material starts to harden. Some patients have a significant gag reflex or a sensation of not being able to breathe enough.

Along with this, the time it takes to let the material set is sometimes irritating for patients and can set back what we accomplish during an appointment. If anything goes wrong with taking the impression, such as improper placement, a bad fit, or if the patient moves, then the impression has to be redone. This takes even more time, and, it's more costly. (A quick side note: it takes about $30 to $50 to get a good upper and lower impression. If we have to redo them, that's more money.) One of my goals is always to cut down on the amount of time the patient has to sit in the chair. It decreases any anxiety they have and increases our productivity. It can also help cut down on cost using a digitally based impression technique.

A final disadvantage to mention is the potential for breaking the impressions. Once the physical impression has been made, if they are dropped, moved, or taken out of the mold too forcefully, they can break. Once they're broken, they can't be used, because gluing them back together doesn't generally provide an accurate enough reflection of the patient's teeth to make a good restoration.

Digital Impressions

Now that we've covered traditional impressions, let's talk about digital impressions. In my practice, we use an intraoral scanner. It's a key element in how we operate and function. It has drastically cut down on inaccurate impressions and is less stressful for our patients. We are able to avoid subjecting patient to gooey materials and trays, and because the impression is digital, there's no fear of breaking, damaging, or losing them. Also, it takes less time for my staff to take an intraoral scan, which means the appointment progresses more quickly, we can get more done, and it takes less time out of the patient's day. We can also see the impressions in real time, so if there is any inaccuracy – or we need a clearer picture – we can immediately retake the scan while the patient is still in the chair.

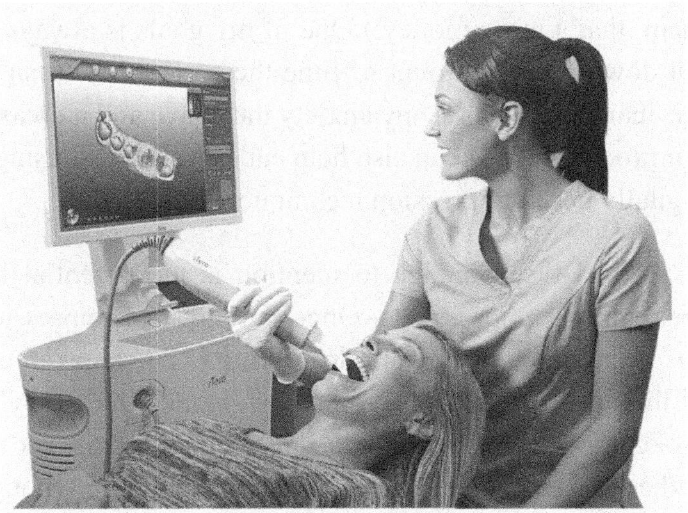

Intraoral scanning of a patient.
Safe, easier on the patient, and more accurate than traditional methods.

Another huge benefit is that because the impressions are electronic, we can send the file to the lab much more quickly than the physical stone impressions can be transported. This decreases turnaround time in processing the impressions and moves the patient's case along more quickly.

Finally, one of the biggest advantages that I've witnessed is the fact that intraoral scans can be saved indefinitely without using up any physical space. This means that, for example, if we create a denture for someone using their digital impression and the denture breaks, we can then use the impressions to create a new denture for them without having to redo the impressions. This saves an incredible amount of work and time, cuts out the need for the patient to come back in, and it's a huge money saver as well.

CAD/CAM Milling and CEREC

CAD/CAM (computer-aided design/computer-aided manufacturing) milling technology, especially the E4D or CEREC system – which is a CAD/CAM product – is becoming more and more popular in dental offices. In some instances, it enables dentists to do chair-side milling of crowns and smaller bridges. Utilizing this technology, we can create the restorations that patients need in one sitting. This is incredibly useful because it decreases turnaround time drastically. Traditional methods – namely creating all restorations in a lab – can take two to three weeks. At most, using the CAD/CAM technology lets us create what we need in less than a week, but, sometimes, as I said above, we can make them almost instantly. It really depends on what the patient wants and needs. Regardless, the time difference is remarkable.

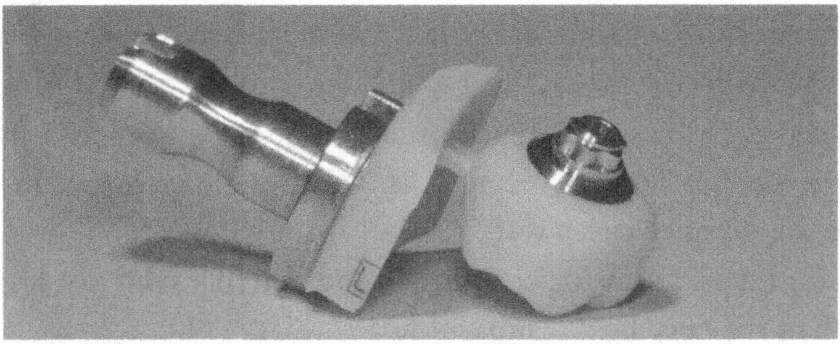

Based on digital scanning, the final restoration can be milled from a solid block of material, creating a stronger restoration.

Also, like with Cone Beam and intraoral scans, this technology improves how we predict the outcomes of our treatment plan and decreases our margin of error significantly. For example, using something like the E4D or CEREC system, dentists can more accurately narrow the edge around where we connect a crown to a patient's tooth, meaning it fits better, functions better, and is less likely to come loose or fall out. It also means that we can decrease the amount of metal, porcelain or various materials used. This improves the aesthetic outcome for the patient.

VIRTUAL SURGERY

Before the advent of digitally guided or virtual surgery, we used traditional 2D x-rays and essentially eyeballed, for example, an implant against the x-ray, saying, "This seems about the right size." We didn't have a true understanding of the full, 3D volumetric of the patient's anatomy in general and specifically around where the implant would be placed. We had to go into surgery and explore placement once we were directly working on the patient. This often led to errors in sizing, positioning – either from a depth, orientation, or an angulation perspective, meaning the angle at which the implant needed to be placed. Although virtual surgery is advancing rapidly in the dental field, as recently as 2015 less than 1% of implant surgery cases were virtually guided, meaning, there is a lot of room for error and more patients who got less than the very best results.

Virtual surgery allows us to harness the advantages of digital dentistry, expanding what we know about patients and their specific needs by using Cone Beam scans and intraoral scans as guides. This enables us to improve patient outcomes by planning beforehand, making a virtual model of our patients and mapping out precisely what needs to be done, and how, before we begin operating. It's much more controlled, which means it leads to a less stressful and unknown operation for us and better results for our patients.

In my own practice, currently more than 95% of my cases are virtually guided. With each one of my patients, I take a CT scan and I use that in conjunction with an intraoral scan. This gives me a clear virtual representation of my patient that I can reference once the patient has left the chair. I can work at my desk and plan out exactly where I need to place an implant, making me confident that the depth, orientation, and angle is perfect before I actually place the implant. This technology also enables us to explore the patient's soft and hard tissue – the gums and jaw bones – helping to determine if changes to the tissue need to be made before operating. Ultimately, when I go into surgery, I'm as confident as possible, knowing that I've used all the technology available to assist me in operating and giving my patient that best result possible.

Using virtual guides also helps cut down on the time it takes to perform oral surgery. The majority of the decisions that need to be made are done beforehand using the virtual model we've created. The virtual guide directs the oral surgeon, allowing them to follow the surgical plan already created and practiced on a computer. This is great for the oral surgeon and also for the patient. It cuts down on the time the patient spends under anesthesia, taking less of a toll on their body and helping them to recover more quickly.

On the Subject of Anesthesia

Since I was just talking about it, I'd like to mention a new digital advancement when it comes to anesthesia. There are now anesthesia machines available that can distribute the proper medications based on the length of time a patient needs to be anesthetized, their body weight, and other factors, using an infusion pump. I utilize these machines which are specifically helpful for surgeries that take a longer amount of time.

These pumps make it easier and safer to get patients to a steady level of anesthetization and keep them there for hours at a time if needed, without using any more medication than is necessary. This means that they don't fluctuate up and down in terms of consciousness. It's much better for the patient because it keeps their heart rate and blood pressure at a safe, steady level. They're comfortable throughout the procedure, not restless, making it easier for the surgeon to do what needs to be done. Additionally, the medications we are able to use are less stressful on the patient, resulting in less post-operative side effects such as nausea and allowing them to come out from the anesthesia quicker and recover faster. In many cases, I'm able to discharge patients within 15 minutes even after a three or four-hour surgery.

A Dental Success Story

I'd like to share the story of one of my patients here. It presents a real-world example and paints a great picture of how digital dentistry can transform the effectiveness of patient treatment.

I had a gentleman come to see me. He needed a full mouth extraction. At 89 years old, he had a compromised medical history. We had a few anesthetic options, but doing local anesthesia wasn't the best choice given his history of anxiety. We could also have sent him to the operating room for general anesthesia, however, this option would have involved going to the hospital and would be harder for him to recover from, especially considering his age and compromised medical status. He decided – and I agreed – that the best option was to use conscious sedation – sometimes referred to as 'twilight' sedation – in the clinic where we had a machine that delivered a consistent, controlled level of medication to keep him calm and comfortable.

We were able to remove all of his upper and lower teeth, reshape his bone, and place a total of 10 implants in less than three hours. Under traditional circumstances, this procedure would take at least four hours or more. I was able to successfully remove his teeth and replace them with implants because I'd planned his entire treatment virtually, utilizing the Cone Beam CT scans and intraoral scans. Because of digital dentistry, we were able to give him his smile back, using the safest sedation option, in a minimal amount of time.

Digital Dentistry in Orthodontics

Digital dentistry is playing a major role in orthodontics. I work with a number of orthodontists who are utilizing intraoral scans and various digital programs to help plan where their patients' teeth need to end up, how they need to move, how quickly they can be moved, and to assist in planning the techniques that will help them accomplish the best outcome for the patients. There are some advanced digital programs that can be used with machines that bend the wires used in braces.

Other digital technologies they use help them plan where the brackets and bands need to go and how they need to be placed, and then the specially-crafted wire is inserted. The orthodontist then already knows that the force the wire places on the teeth, teamed with the brackets and bands, is going to move the teeth at the right speed and get them into the right position because he's used virtual models ahead of time. This cuts down significantly on the time it takes to put the braces on, make the needed changes during each phase of movement, and it can ultimately help cut down on the length of time the patient is in the chair per appointment and the total length of treatment time the braces need to stay on. Many orthodontists I work closely with are also utilizing 3D printers to print up models of the patient's teeth at each stage of the treatment plan, enabling them to make guides and trays for patients to utilize in between the stages to keep the teeth where they need to be.

The newer trend in orthodontics is to virtually plan the tooth movements. Then break the desired movements into steps that is tolerable for the biology of the human body to accept. These steps are then printed into clear retainers that the patient sequentially wears over several months to achieve the desired movement. This process works well and is becoming the go to option for people who do not want traditional brackets and wires. In my opinion it is critical that before the patient begins a trained orthodontist still physically sees the patient to ensure that this is the correct treatment.

3D Printers

This is a good time to talk about 3D printers, which are the companion technology to 3D scans. These printers really came from the prototyping community, people who were just looking to print up small models of things they needed or were working on. They've gotten bigger and more widely used in a number of industries since they first came onto the scene, but the dental field has really taken hold of the 3D printing technology and incorporated it beautifully into the mix of digital and technological advancements used to treat patients. As noted previously, orthodontists print up models, guides, and trays for themselves and for patients. In my case, as an oral surgeon, I utilize our 3D printer to print up a real-life model which I can use as a surgical guide before I operate, allowing me to visualize and plan every step of a surgery.

3D printers have come down in cost and their accuracy has improved immensely in the past four years or so.

These changes are so significant that I can count on one hand the number of orthodontists I work with who don't now use a 3D printer.

These printers are incredibly advanced, reshaping our ability to design and produce restorations of teeth that are the perfect shape and color for implant patients. There are some amazing digital libraries of teeth that provide crucial models we can use to make teeth that fit almost seamlessly with a patient's other teeth. To be fair, it's still a difficult task, even with these 3D printers, to make perfect teeth because there are so many nuances in shape and shading when it comes to teeth. But the improvement over using traditional x-ray technology is remarkable.

The Importance of Being Well-Versed in Digital Dentistry

I believe that innovation is the key to progress; if you don't learn and adapt to the latest technology, you will inevitably be surpassed. Digital dentistry is really the latest in a line of advancements the dental field has embraced. For patients, I believe it's important to seek out an oral surgeon that is, well-versed in digital dentistry. This comes from education and practice. It's important for patients to find an oral surgeon that is constantly looking for the best techniques and treatments, options that enable them to provide the very best care and thus give patients the very best results, both structurally and aesthetically.

Every patient is different, and every case is unique in some way. Digital options allow us to explore new ways to give every patient exactly the treatment they need and the outcome they want. The flexibility that digital dentistry offers lends itself to helping us give the most personalized care.

The Patient Always Comes First

Patient safety, comfort, and satisfaction are at the core of everything I do. Digital dentistry helps me check off all three of these things. Using the Cone Beam scanner first – which, again, gives me the most information with the least amount of radiation exposure to my patient – is the beginning of the process. Using the intraoral scans and the 3D printer makes it easy for me to thoroughly plan the course of treatment for the patient, keeping in mind that it helps me cut down the length of time I'm operating on my patient, which is safer for them and makes the recovery process easier afterward. All the digital elements I use in my practice boost my accuracy, my confidence, and that, in turn, makes the patient feel more assured and ultimately more satisfied once their case is finished.

I genuinely believe that when a patient is looking for an oral surgeon he or she should look for the doctor that has their best interest at heart and is willing to utilize every option available to give them the very best care. In my personal experience, digital dentistry plays a vital role in how effective the doctor is and the level and quality of care that he or she can offer.

Digital Dentistry Investment

There are a number of reasons why I feel that many dentists, oral surgeons, and other doctors aren't jumping into digital dentistry. The number one concern is the expense. None of the digital options I've talked about are cheap. They are, in fact, rather expensive endeavors. I believe, from what I've seen and heard, that many doctors are afraid to make these major investments. Especially because it is new technology, and with the rapid and ever-changing advancements that occur in technology, the concern is that the technology they invest in will become outdated fairly quickly. Eventually, more money to update the technology they've invested in will be necessary. The thing to note with this is that digital dentistry is, in fact, an investment. It costs money to provide high-quality dentistry. And as with most investments, the dividends are paid out over time, with each patient, when we can offer better, safer, and more accurate care with every case we work on.

Ultimately, the upfront cost of the technology, in my opinion, more than pays for itself in two primary ways. First, we save time and money because we are able to better plan treatments and accomplish our end goal more rapidly. Second, and perhaps the more important way – at least for me – is the repayment I get when a patient sees their new smile and is overjoyed. It's not a financial repayment, but it's a big part of why I use digital dentistry.

Another reason that many practices aren't using digital dentistry is the time commitment it requires to learn to use the new technology. Whether it's a new doctor that's trying to keep their head above water and pay off loans for their new practice, or an older doctor who's been treating patients with the same techniques for his entire career, using digital dentistry takes a serious commitment to educating oneself in the various technologies and aspects of using digital guides to aid them in the treatment process. Coupled with the new advancements and the different technologies available, when a doctor decides to implement digital dentistry into their practice, it requires constantly updating oneself on the newest and latest information regarding each type of technology. This is another investment, one of time, and it's a considerable one. But in the end, the time I spent educating myself has paid for itself over and over with every case I've completed successfully.

The reality is that these concerns over digital dentistry are holding a lot of doctors and practices back from offering their patients the best care, by using the latest technology available. However, I do see that the numbers of surgeons performing guided surgeries is increasing because more and more dentists and doctors recognize the advantages. When it comes to intraoral scanners, I'd say that probably at least a quarter of oral surgeons are now using them. And when it comes to Cone Beam scanners, they are basically a standard of care at this point among oral surgeons.

The Mountain Biker Story

I'd like to share one more patient story with you. Her case is another great example of how digital dentistry works in real life.

A young woman who was pregnant came to see me. She'd been mountain biking in Colorado and had a severe accident. She'd gone over the top of her handlebars, fractured her lower jaw in two places, and broke her two upper front teeth. The other four front anterior teeth were also quite loose. We were able to take Cone Beam scans before we began working to repair her jaw.

While her jaws were healing, we were able to create a digital model of her jaws and teeth, allowing us to plan how to remove the broken teeth and also where to accurately put in implants, so that we could have her temporary teeth ready right away. As soon as her jaw had healed, we placed her implants and her temporary teeth. She was able to return to work in a very short period of time, and the ultimate result she got was a beautiful smile.

A Final Note

In concluding this chapter, I feel it's important to explain a little bit about my experience with digital dentistry and why I'm passionate about staying up-to-date on the latest advancements.

I completed my oral & maxillofacial surgery residency in 2008. At that time, digital dentistry was still a new concept. There was some implant planning being done digitally. The first orthognathic cases were performed digitally shortly after that. Most of my experience with digital dentistry stems from my time in the Air Force, where I was in charge of facial traumas in Germany, working on soldiers that were coming out of Iraq and Afghanistan.

Working on these cases, employing the digital options that were available, allowed me to give my fellow soldiers the best care possible. I was able to map out a plan that would get them treated and rehabbed from their injuries as quickly as possible. The knowledge and experienced that I gained overseas was the impetus to transition into doing more digital implant dentistry when I got home.

My experience working on injured soldiers and seeing the benefits of digital dentistry in their cases, then employing those same techniques in my current practice, is what keeps me pushing to learn and utilize the latest digital and technological advancements.

At the end of the day, it all comes down to this: I want to give my patients the very best care. I want to treat each one like I treated the injured soldiers. I want each of my patients to feel safe, to feel confident, and to understand that every step of their treatment is carefully planned and that I have a backup plan as well. When their treatment is complete, seeing my patients smile, sometimes for the first time in a long time, I know that I've fulfilled my purpose. This is why I use digital dentistry, and that is why I love what I do.

About Curtis Hayes, DDS

Coal Creek Oral Surgery and Dental Implant Center
www.CoalCreekOMS.com

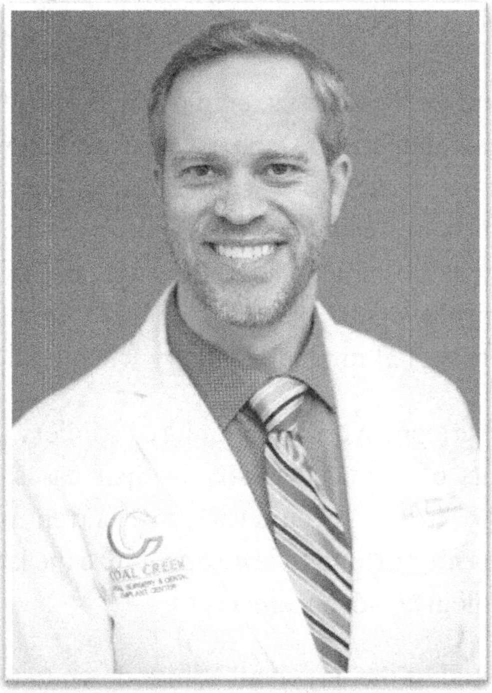

Dr. Curtis Hayes offers exceptional skill and experience to his patients seeking restorative and cosmetic dental care. A board-certified oral surgeon, Dr. Hayes completed a Bachelor of Science in Biochemistry at the United States Air Force Academy before attending the University of Colorado School of Dentistry, where he graduated *magna cum laude* in 2003.

Dr. Hayes served as a dentist at Lackland Air Force Base before continuing his education in oral surgery at

Wilford Hall Medical Center in San Antonio. He also served as the Chief of Oral and Maxillofacial Surgery at Ramstein Air Force Base in Germany, where he was named 2013 US Air Force Dentist of the Year for his care to wounded service members serving in Africa and the Middle East.

A skilled educator who has contributed to many peer-reviewed journals, Dr. Hayes has also served as the Director of Oral and Maxillofacial Surgery for the Advanced Education in General Dentistry Program. He is a member of the Colorado Society of Oral and Maxillofacial Surgeons as well as the American and Colorado Dental Associations, and is a Fellow of the American Association of Oral and Maxillofacial Surgeons and a Diplomate of the American Board of Oral and Maxillofacial Surgeons.

Dr. Hayes believes in helping to educate the public about dental care as well. He has appeared on both Colorado and National Public Radio, given interviews to the *Boulder Daily Camera*, and appeared on the USAF AOG "Checkpoints" with expert advice on opioid use in dental treatments.

Dr. Hayes has participated locally for more than twenty years as an adult leader in the Boy Scouts of America and has worked on missions to the Peruvian Amazon Basin and South Africa. He also volunteers as a clinical instructor at the University of Colorado School of Dental Medicine. Dr. Hayes and his team pride themselves on being reassuring, kind, and compassionate in addition to highly skilled.

Made in United States
Orlando, FL
10 November 2026

90498881R00118